KETO DIET COOKBOOK FOR WOMEN OVER 50

251 HEALTHY, DELICIOUS AND EFFECTIVE RECIPES FOR FASTER WEIGHT LOSS THAT WILL HELP YOU FEEL GOOD, STAY FAB AND ENERGETIC AT 50

Gracelynn Rogers

Table of Contents

INTRODUCTION

Over the age of 50, it is hard to maintain good health and shed extra weight, especially for women. Either they are experiencing menopause, having more time to eat and socializing, losing weight after 50 is not easy.

The ketogenic diet provides the body with premium fuel in the form of fats that make you fitter and younger with the energy of a twenty-year-old, and the best part, it lasts longer than carb fuel.

By following the ketogenic diet, you can lose all the unwanted weight without ever stepping foot in a gym, without any meal portion control or counting calories. The ketogenic diet has proven to work for people with all types of background and health issues like having blood sugar issues, obesity, post-pregnancy, people having food addictions, suffering from emotional eating, etc.

Adaptation to ketosis can be tough, and you will need time to adjust to the changes. It is normal, and everyone faces troubles in adapting to any new dietary plan. However, here are some steps to help you in transiting into the ketogenic diet plan perfectly. Just remember that it does require time, and you will have to give yourself a little space to adjust to the restrictions. It won't happen overnight, so don't be disheartened and stay motivated!

The most basic mistake that many keto dieters make is that they don't gain enough knowledge before starting the diet. Therefore, the most important step is to learn the small differences that make a huge difference. Understand what keto-friendly foods are what foods are not meant for ketosis at all. For example, a lot of apple does not eat an apple because it has many carbs. However, if you have a medium or a small-sized apple, then you are good to have it. As long as it remains within your carb limit, it is keto-friendly. You can also eat an apple a day (depending on the size), but you need to remember ketosis's essence and take your carbs from energetic sources like protein and healthy fats. Once you can understand the difference between non-keto and keto-friendly foods, you will notice that ketosis is not that tough after all.

The best way to transit in ketosis is to keep track of your carbs. This might seem annoying at first, but you will gradually see how helpful it is, and you will eventually understand the importance of calculating the net carbs per day. It is extremely crucial, and usually, people overlook this issue quite easily. However, if you want to settle into ketosis perfectly, it is best to keep track of your net carbs.

Mindful eating is a very important step towards transition into ketosis. Your caloric intake has a huge impact on your weight loss. The more calories you take, the harder it gets to lose the stubborn, stored fat. A keto calculator can be extremely helpful in this matter, though. You can calculate your caloric intake on the go and limit your food intake accordingly. Also, before you pick something to eat, you can instantly calculate the calories you will take. This is known as mindful eating, knowing what you are eating and how it will affect you.

Ketosis is all about gaining knowledge and getting into the habit of mindful eating. Once you know what you are eating and how much it has to offer to you, you will gradually see major changes in your overall diet routine. You will also find yourself adjusting to ketosis much easier.

CHAPTER 1: BENEFITS OF KETO DIET FOR WOMEN OVER 50

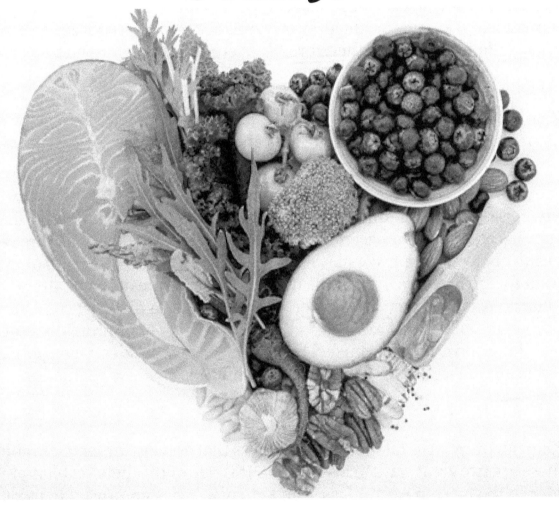

The Keto diet has been proven to have many benefits for people over 50. Here are some of the best.

Strengthens bones

When people get older, their bones weaken. At 50, your bones are likely not as strong as they used to be. However, you can keep them in really good condition. Consuming milk to get calcium cannot do enough to strengthen your bones. What you can do is to make use of the Keto diet as it is low in toxins. Toxins negatively affect the absorption of nutrients, and so with this, your bones can take in all they need.

Eradicates inflammation

Few things are worse than the pain from an inflamed joint or muscle. Arthritis, for instance, can be extremely difficult to bear. When you follow the ketosis diet, the production of cytokines will be reduced. Cytokines cause inflammation, and therefore, their eradication will reduce it.

It eradicates nutrients deficiency

Keto focuses on consuming exactly what you need. If you use a great Keto plan, your body will lack no nutrients and will not suffer any deficiency.

Reduced hunger

The reason we find it difficult to stick to diets is hunger. It doesn't matter your age; diets do not become easier. We may have a mental picture of the healthy body we want. We may even have clear visuals of the kind of life we want to lead once free from unhealthy living, but none of that matters when hunger enters the scene. However, the Keto diet is a diet that combats this problem. The Keto diet focuses on consuming plenty of proteins. Proteins are filling and do not let you feel hungry too easily. Besides, when your carb levels are reduced, your appetite takes a hit. It is a win-win situation.

Weight loss

Keto not only burns fat, but it also reduces that craving for food. Combined, these are two great ways to lose weight. It is one of the diets that has proven to help the most in weight loss. The Keto diet has been proven to be one of the best ways to burn stubborn belly fat while keeping yourself revitalized and healthy.

Reduces blood sugar and insulin

After 50, monitoring blood sugar can be a real struggle. Drastically, cutting down on carbs reduces both insulin levels and blood sugar levels. It means that the Keto diet will benefit millions as many people struggle with insulin complications and high blood sugar levels. It has been proven to help when some people embark on Keto, and they cut up to half of the carbs they consume. It's a treasure for those with diabetes and insulin resistance. A study was carried out on people with type 2 diabetes. After cutting down on carbs, within six months, 95 percent of people could reduce or stop using their glucose-lowering medication.

Lower levels of triglycerides

Many people do not know what triglycerides are. Triglycerides are molecules of fat in your blood. They are known to circulate in the bloodstream and can be very dangerous. High levels of triglycerides can cause heart failures and heart diseases. However, Keto is known to reduce these levels.

Reduces acne

Although young people mostly suffer acne, there are cases of people above 50 having it. Moreover, Keto is not only for persons after 50. Acne is not only caused by blocked pores. There are quite some things proven to drive it. One of these things is your blood sugar. When you consume processed and refined carbs, it affects gut bacteria and results in blood sugar levels fluctuation. When the gut bacteria and sugar levels are affected, the skin suffers. However, when you embark on the Keto diet, you cut off on carbs intake, which means that in the very first place, your gut bacteria will not be affected, thereby cutting off that avenue to develop.

Increases HDL levels

HDL refers to high-density lipoprotein. When your HDL levels are compared to your LDL levels and are not found low, your risk of developing heart disease is lowered. It is great for persons over 50 as heart diseases suddenly become more probable. Eating fats and reducing your intake of carbohydrates is one of the most certain ways to increase your high-density lipoprotein levels.

Reduces LDL levels

High levels of LDL can be very problematic when you attain 50. It is because LDL refers to bad cholesterol. People with high levels of this cholesterol are more likely to get heart attacks. When you reduce the number of carbs you consume, you will increase the size of bad LDL particles. However, this will reduce the total LDL particles as they would have increased in size. Smaller LDL particles have been linked to heart diseases, while larger ones have been proven to have lower risks attached.

May help combat cancer

I termed this under 'may' because research on this is not as extensive and conclusive as we would like it to be. However, there is proof supporting it. Firstly, it helps reduce the levels of blood sugar, which lowers insulin complications, which in turn reduces the risk of developing cancers related to insulin levels. Besides, Keto places more oxidative stress on cancer cells than normal cells, making it great for chemotherapy. The risk of developing cancer after fifty is still existent, and so, Keto is a lifesaver.

May lower blood pressure

High blood pressure plagues adults much more than it do young ones. Once you attain 50, you must monitor your blood pressure rates. Reduction in the intake of carbohydrates is a proven way to lower your blood pressure. When you cut down on your carbs and lower your blood sugar levels, you greatly reduce your chances of getting other diseases.

Combats metabolic syndrome

As you grow older, you may find that you struggle to control your blood sugar level. Metabolic syndrome is another condition that has been proven to influence diabetes and heart disease development. The symptoms associated with metabolic syndrome include but are not limited to high triglycerides, obesity, high blood sugar level, and low levels of high-density lipoprotein cholesterol.

However, you will find that reducing your level of carbohydrate intake greatly affects this. You will improve your health and majorly attack all the above-listed symptoms. Keto diet helps to fight against metabolic syndrome, which is a big win.

Great for the heart

People over the age of 50 have been proven to have more chances of developing heart diseases. Keto diet has been proven to be great for the heart. As the good cholesterol levels rises and bad cholesterol levels decreases, you will find that partaking in the Keto diet proves extremely beneficial for your health.

May reduce seizure risks

When you change your intake levels, the combination of protein, fat, and carbs, as we explained before, your body will go into ketosis. Ketosis has been proven to reduce seizure levels in people who have epilepsy. When they do not respond to treatment, the ketosis treatment is used. It has been done for decades.

Combats brain disorders

Keto doesn't end there, and it also combats Alzheimer's and Parkinson's disease. Some parts of your brain can only burn glucose, and so, your body needs it. If you do not consume carbs, your lover will make use of protein to produce glucose. Your brain can also burn ketones. Ketones are formed when your carb level is very low. With this, the ketogenic diet has been used f r plenty of years to treat epilepsy in children who aren't responding to drugs. For adults, it can work the same magic as it is now being linked to treating Alzheimer's and Parkinson's disease

CHAPTER 2. SMOOTHIES RECIPES

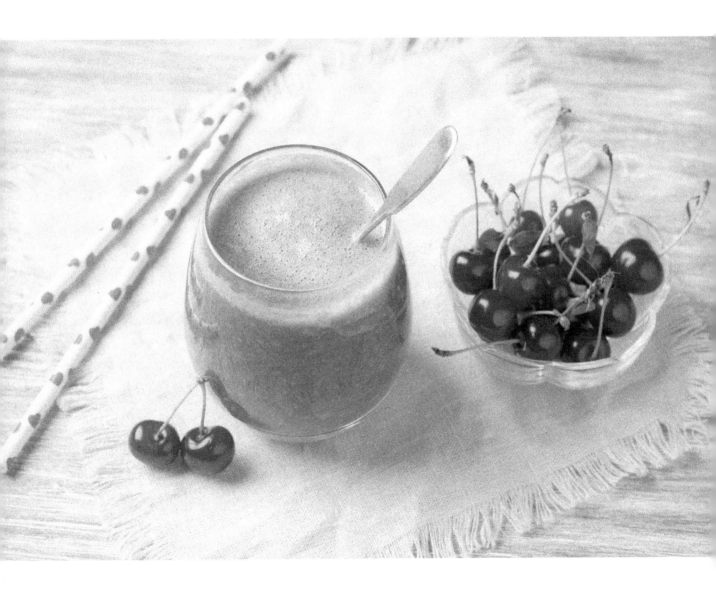

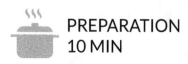 **PREPARATION**
10 MIN

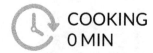 **COOKING**
0 MIN

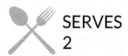 **SERVES**
2

1. RED FESTIVE SMOOTHIE

INGREDIENTS

- ¾ C. raw red beets, chopped
- 4 frozen strawberries
- 2-3 drops liquid stevia
- 1½ C. unsweetened almond milk
- ½ C. ice cubes

DIRECTIONS

At high-speed blender, mix all the ingredients and pulse until smooth.

Fill into 2 serving glasses and serve immediately.

Nutrition: 66 Calories 9g Carbohydrates 2g Protein

PREPARATION
10 MIN
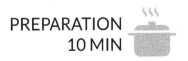

COOKING
0 MIN
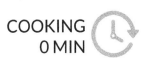

SERVES
2

2. PRETTY PINK SMOOTHIE

INGREDIENTS

- ½ c. fresh strawberries, hulled
- 8-10 fresh basil leaves
- 3-4 drops liquid stevia
- ½ C. plain Greek yogurt
- 1 C. unsweetened almond milk
- ¼ C. ice cubes

DIRECTIONS

In a high-speed blender, incorporate all the ingredients and pulse until smooth.

Pour into 2 serving glasses and serve.

Nutrition: 75 Calories 8g Carbohydrates 4.3g Protein

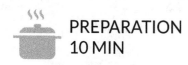

PREPARATION
10 MIN

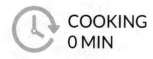

COOKING
0 MIN

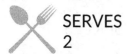

SERVES
2

3. GOLDEN CHAI LATTE SMOOTHIE

INGREDIENTS

- 2 tbsp. chia seeds
- 1 tbsp. ground turmeric
- 1 tsp. ground cinnamon
- 1 tsp. ground ginger
- ¼ tsp. ground cardamom
- Pinch of ground black pepper
- 2 tbsp. MCT oil
- 2 tsp. stevia powder
- 1¾ C. unsweetened almond milk
- ¼ C. ice cubes

DIRECTIONS

With a high-speed blender, add all the ingredients and pulse until smooth.

Transfer into 2 serving glasses and serve immediately.

Nutrition: 178 Calories 8.5g Carbohydrates 2.7g Protein

PREPARATION
10 MIN
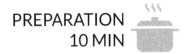

4. VELVETY CHOCOLATE SMOOTHIE

COOKING
0 MIN
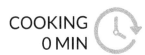

SERVES
2
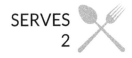

INGREDIENTS

- ¼ C. cacao powder
- ¼ C. almond butter
- 1 tbsp. almonds
- 5-6 drops liquid stevia
- 1 C. unsweetened almond milk
- ½ C. unsweetened coconut milk
- ¼ C. ice cubes

DIRECTIONS

Using a high-speed blender, add all the ingredients and pulse until smooth.

Transfer into 2 serving glasses and serve immediately.

Nutrition: 110 Calories 7.5g Carbohydrates 3.8g Protein

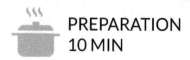

PREPARATION
10 MIN

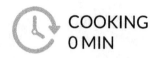

COOKING
0 MIN

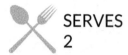

SERVES
2

5. CREAMY TEXTURED SMOOTHIE

INGREDIENTS

- ½ C. avocado
- 3 tbsp. Monk fruit sweetener
- 2 tbsp. natural creamy peanut butter
- 2 tbsp. cacao powder
- 1½ C. unsweetened almond milk
- ½ C. ice, crushed

DIRECTIONS

Process all the ingredients until smooth.

Pour into glasses and serve.

Nutrition: 222 Calories 10g Carbohydrates 5.9g Protein

6. LATTE BREAKFAST SMOOTHIE

PREPARATION
10 MIN
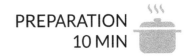

COOKING
0 MIN
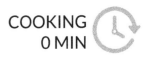

SERVES
2
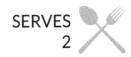

INGREDIENTS

- ▶ 1 scoop unflavored collagen powder
- ▶ 1 tbsp. MCT oil
- ▶ 1 tbsp. chia seeds
- ▶ 1-2 tbsp. Swerve
- ▶ ½ tsp. ground cinnamon
- ▶ 12 oz. cold brewed coffee
- ▶ 1 C. unsweetened almond milk

DIRECTIONS

In blender, add all the ingredients and pulse until smooth.

Transfer into 2 serving glasses and serve immediately.

Nutrition: 144 Calories 4g Carbohydrates 15.2g Protein

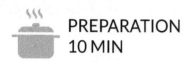

PREPARATION
10 MIN

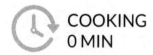

COOKING
0 MIN

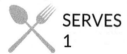

SERVES
1

7. SMOOTHIE IN A BOWL

INGREDIENTS

- Almond milk (.5 cup)
- Spinach (1 cup)
- Heavy cream (2 tbsp.)
- Low-carb protein powder (1 scoop)
- Coconut oil (1 tbsp.)
- Ice (2 cubes)
- **For Toppings:**
- Walnuts (4)
- Raspberries (4)
- Chia seeds 1 tsp.)

- Shredded coconut (1 tbsp.)

DIRECTIONS

Add a cup of spinach to your high-speed blender. Pour in the cream, almond milk, ice, and coconut oil.

Blend for a few seconds until it has an even consistency, and all ingredients are well combined. Empty the goodies into a serving dish.

Arrange your toppings or give them a toss and mix them together. Of course, you can make it pretty and alternate the strips of toppings.

Nutrition: 35g Protein 35g Fats 570 Calories

8. STRAWBERRY & RHUBARB PIE SMOOTHIE

PREPARATION
12 MIN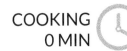

COOKING
0 MIN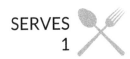

SERVES
1

INGREDIENTS

- Almond butter (2 tbsp. or 1 oz. almonds)
- Medium rhubarb stalks (1.8 oz. - 1-2 stalks)
- Medium strawberries (2-4 or 1.4 oz.)
- Large organic/free-range egg (1)
- Coconut milk - full-fat cream (2 tbsp.)
- Unsweetened almond milk (.5 cup)
- Vanilla bean (1) or pure vanilla bean extract (.5 tsp.)
- Ginger root powder (.5 tsp.) or freshly grated ginger root (1 tsp.)
- Liquid stevia extract – vanilla or clear (3-6 drops)

DIRECTIONS

Combine each of the ingredients into a blender.

Pulse and enjoy when smooth.

Nutrition: 14.2g Protein 31.8g Fats 392 Calories

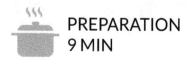

PREPARATION
9 MIN

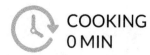

COOKING
0 MIN

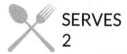

SERVES
2

9. STRAWBERRY SMOOTHIES

INGREDIENTS

- Almonds (8)
- Whey protein powder (1.5 scoops)
- Large strawberries (2)
- Unsweetened almond milk (16 oz.)
- Cubes of ice (6)

DIRECTIONS

Add all of the fixings in your blender.

Wait for the ice to break apart.

Serve in two 10-oz. chilled glasses.

Nutrition: 18.9g Protein 6.6g Fats 156.8 Calories

PREPARATION
7 MIN
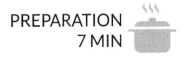

COOKING
0 MIN
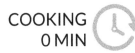

SERVES
1
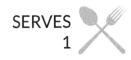

10. VANILLA FAT-BURNING SMOOTHIE

INGREDIENTS

- Mascarpone full-fat cheese (.5 cup)
- Large egg yolks (2)
- Water (.25 cup)
- Coconut oil (1 tbsp.)
- Ice cubes (4)
- Liquid stevia (3 drops)
- Pure vanilla extract (.5 tsp.)
- Optional Topping: Whipped cream

DIRECTIONS

Combine all of the fixings in a blender. Blend until smooth.

Add the whipped cream for a special treat, but add the carbs if any.

Nutrition: 64g Fats 12g Protein 651 Calories

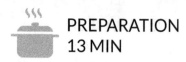

PREPARATION
13 MIN

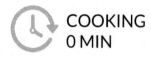

COOKING
0 MIN

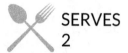

SERVES
2

11. ALMOND & BLUEBERRY SMOOTHIE

INGREDIENTS

- Unsweetened almond milk (16 oz.)
- Heavy cream (4 oz.)
- Stevia (to taste)
- Whey vanilla isolate powder (1 scoop)
- Frozen unsweetened blueberries (.25 cup)

DIRECTIONS

Throw all of the fixings into a blender.

Mix until smooth.

Serve it up in a couple of chilled glasses.

Nutrition: 15g Protein 25g Fats 302 Calories

12. AVOCADO SMOOTHIE

PREPARATION
5 MIN
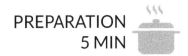

COOKING
0 MIN
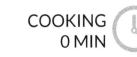

SERVES
1

INGREDIENTS

- Avocado (1)
- Ice cubes (6)
- EZ-Sweetz sweetener (6 drops)
- Unsweetened almond milk (3 oz.)
- Coconut cream (3 oz.)

DIRECTIONS

Slice the avocado lengthwise. Remove the seeds and the skin.

Toss the avocado with the rest of the fixings into the blender.

Toss in the ice cubes and blend until the smoothie is creamy smooth.

Nutrition: 6g Protein 58g Fats 587 Calories

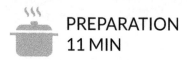
PREPARATION
11 MIN

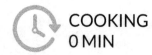
COOKING
0 MIN

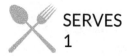
SERVES
1

13. AVOCADO MINT GREEN SMOOTHIE

INGREDIENTS

- ▸ Avocado (3-4 oz. or .5 of 1)
- ▸ Cilantro (3 sprigs)
- ▸ Mint leaves (5-6 large)
- ▸ Vanilla extract (.25 tsp.)
- ▸ Lime juice (1 squeeze)
- ▸ Sweetener of your choice (as desired)
- ▸ Full-fat coconut milk (.75 cup)
- ▸ Almond milk (.5 cup)
- ▸ Crushed ice (1.5 cups)

DIRECTIONS

Portion each of the ingredients into the blender.

Puree it using the low-speed setting.

Toss in the ice and mix. Serve in a cold mug.

Nutrition: 23g Fats 1g Protein 221 Calories

PREPARATION
16 MIN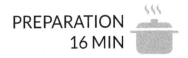

COOKING
0 MIN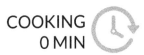

SERVES
2

14. BANANA BREAD - BLUEBERRY SMOOTHIE

INGREDIENTS

- Blueberries (.25 cup)
- Chia seeds (1 tbsp.)
- Liquid stevia (10 drops)
- MCT oil (2 tbsp.)
- Golden flaxseed meal (3 tbsp.)
- Vanilla unsweetened coconut milk (2 cups)
- Xanthan gum (.25 tsp.)
- Banana extract (1.5 tsp.)
- Ice cubes (2-3)

DIRECTIONS

Mix each of the fixings into a blender.

Set aside for few minutes for the seeds and flax to absorb some of the liquid.

Pulse for one or two minutes until well combined.

Add the ice to your preference.

Nutrition: 23.3g Fats 3.1g Protein 270 Calories

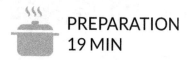

PREPARATION
19 MIN

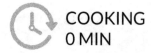

COOKING
0 MIN

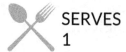

SERVES
1

15. BLACKBERRY CHEESECAKE SMOOTHIE

INGREDIENTS

- ▸ Extra-virgin coconut oil (1 tbsp.)
- ▸ Fresh/frozen blackberries (.5 cup)
- ▸ Water (.5 cup)
- ▸ Coconut milk/heavy whipping cream (.25 cup)
- ▸ Full-fat cream cheese (.25 cup)
- ▸ Sugar-free vanilla extract (.5 tsp.)
- ▸ Liquid stevia (3 to 5 drops as desired)

DIRECTIONS

Arrange all of the fixings in the blender.

Pulse until it's smooth and frothy.

Add a few ice cubes and enjoy it in a chilled glass.

Nutrition: 6g Protein 53g Fats 515 Calories

PREPARATION
16 MIN
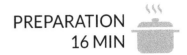

16. BLUEBERRY YOGURT SMOOTHIE

COOKING
0 MIN
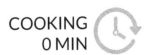

SERVES
2

INGREDIENTS

- Blueberries (10)
- Yogurt (.5 cup)
- Vanilla extract (.5 tsp.)
- Coconut milk (1 cup)
- Stevia (as desired)

DIRECTIONS

Add all of the fixings into a blender. Mix well.

When creamy smooth, pour into two chilled mugs and enjoy.

Nutrition: 2g Protein 5g Fats 70 Calories

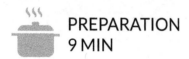

PREPARATION
9 MIN

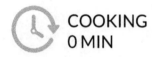

COOKING
0 MIN

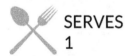

SERVES
1

17. CHOCOLATE & CINNAMON SMOOTHIE

INGREDIENTS

- Coconut milk (.75 cup)
- Ripened avocado (.5 of 1)
- Cinnamon powder (1 tsp.)
- Unsweetened cacao powder (2 tsp.)
- Vanilla extract (.25 tsp.)
- Stevia (as desired)
- Optional: Coconut oil (1 tsp.)

DIRECTIONS

Blend all of the above fixings and combine well.

Pour and serve when ready.

Nutrition: 3g Protein 30g Fats 300 Calories

PREPARATION
11 MIN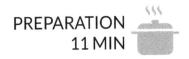

COOKING
0 MIN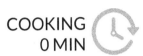

SERVES
1

18. CINNAMON ROLL SMOOTHIE

INGREDIENTS

- Vanilla protein powder (2 tbsp.)
- Flax meal (1 tsp.)
- Almond milk (1 cup)
- Vanilla extract (.25 tsp.)
- Sweetener (4 tsp.)
- Cinnamon (.5 tsp.)
- Ice (1 cup)

DIRECTIONS

Mix all of the fixings in a blender.

Lastly, empty the ice.

Blend using the high setting for 30 seconds or until thickened.

Nutrition: 26.5g Protein 3.25g Fats 145 Calories

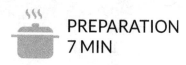

PREPARATION
7 MIN

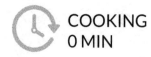

COOKING
0 MIN

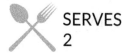

SERVES
2

19. CUCUMBER SPINACH SMOOTHIES

INGREDIENTS

- Ice cubes (6)
- Your choice of sweetener (to taste)
- Coconut milk (.75 cup)
- MCT oil (2 tbsp.)
- Cucumber (2.5 oz.)
- Spinach (2 handfuls)
- Coconut milk (1 cup)
- Xanthan gum (.25 tsp.)

DIRECTIONS

Cream the coconut milk: This is a simple process. Chill coconut milk overnight. The next morning, open then scoop out the coconut milk that has solidified. Don't shake the can before opening. Discard the liquids.

Add all of the ingredients, save the ice cubes, to the blender and blend using the low speed until pureed. Thin with water as needed.

Stir in the ice cubes and blend until the smoothie reaches your desired consistency.

Nutrition: 10g Protein 32g Fats 330 Calories

20. DELIGHTFUL CHOCOLATE SMOOTHIE

PREPARATION
6 MIN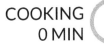

COOKING
0 MIN

SERVES
1

INGREDIENTS

- Large eggs (2)
- Extra-virgin coconut oil (1 tbsp.)
- Almond or coconut butter (1-2 tbsp.)
- Heavy whipping cream (.25 cup)
- Chia seeds (1-2 tbsp.)
- Cinnamon (.5 tsp.)
- Stevia extract (3-5 drops)
- Plain or chocolate whey protein (.25 cup)
- Unsweetened cacao powder (1 tbsp.)
- Water (.25 cup)
- Vanilla extract (.5 tsp.)
- Ice (.5 cup)

DIRECTIONS

Beat eggs with the rest of fixings into a blender.

Pulse until frothy.

Add to a chilled glass and enjoy.

Nutrition: 34.5g Protein 46g Fats 570 Calories

CHAPTER 3. BREAKFAST RECIPES

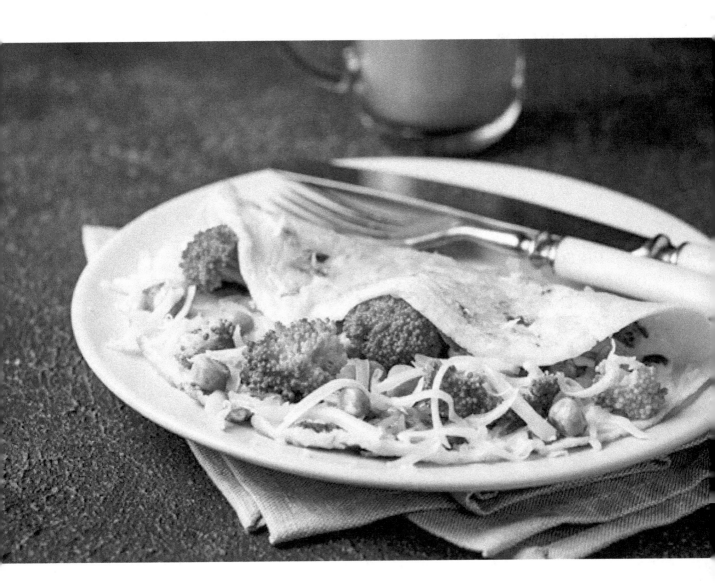

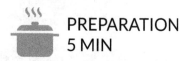

PREPARATION
5 MIN

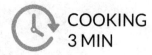

COOKING
3 MIN

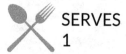

SERVES
1

21. TASTY OMELET CHAFFLES

INGREDIENTS

- 2 eggs, lightly beaten
- 1 tbsp bell pepper, chopped
- 1 tbsp ham, chopped
- 2 tbsp cheddar cheese, shredded
- 2 tbsp almond milk
- Pepper
- Salt

DIRECTIONS

Preheat the waffle maker.

In a bowl, whisk eggs. Add remaining ingredients and stir well.

Coat waffle maker with cooking spray.

Fill in batter in the hot waffle maker and cook for 2-3 minutes or until set.

Serve and enjoy.

Nutrition: 304 Calories 22g Fat 12g Carbohydrates

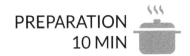

PREPARATION
10 MIN

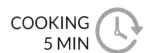

COOKING
5 MIN

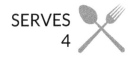

SERVES
4

22. BREAKFAST OMELET

INGREDIENTS

- 4 large eggs
- 2 oz cheddar cheese, shredded
- 8 olives, pitted
- 2 tbsp butter
- 2 tbsp olive oil
- 1 tsp herb de Provence
- 1/2 tsp salt

DIRECTIONS

Whisk eggs in a bowl with salt, olives, herb de Provence, and olive oil.

Melt butter in a large pan over medium heat.

Pour egg mixture into the hot pan and spread evenly.

Cover and cook for 3 minutes or until omelet lightly golden brown.

Flip omelet to the other side and cook for 2 minutes more.

Serve and enjoy.

Nutrition: 251 Calories 22g Fat 1.1g Carbohydrates

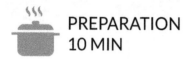

PREPARATION
10 MIN

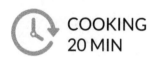

COOKING
20 MIN

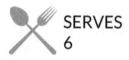

SERVES
6

23. MEXICAN FRITTATA

INGREDIENTS

- 8 eggs, scrambled
- 1/2 cup salsa
- 2 tsp taco seasoning, homemade
- 1/2 lb. ground beef
- 1/2 cup cheddar cheese, grated
- 2 tbsp green onion, chopped
- 1/3 lb. tomatoes, sliced
- 1 small green pepper, chopped
- 1 tbsp olive oil
- 1/4 tsp salt

DIRECTIONS

Preheat the oven to 375 F.

Cook oil in a pan over medium heat.

Fry beef until browned.

Add salsa and taco seasoning and stir to coat.

Remove meat from the pan and place on a plate.

Add green pepper to the pan and cook for a few minutes.

Return meat to the pan along with green onion and tomato.

Add scrambled eggs on top then sprinkle with grated cheese.

Bake for 20-25 minutes.

Nutrition: 227 Calories 13.8g Fat 4g Carbohydrates

24. PROTEIN WAFFLE

PREPARATION
5 MIN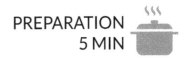

COOKING
10 MIN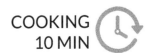

SERVES
2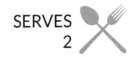

INGREDIENTS

- 1 egg, lightly beaten
- 1 tbsp almond milk
- 1 scoop protein powder
- 1/4 tsp baking powder, gluten-free
- 1 tbsp butter, melted
- 1/4 tsp salt

DIRECTIONS

Incorporate all ingredients in a bowl.

Spray waffle maker with cooking spray.

Pour half of the mix in waffle maker and cook until golden brown. Repeat.

Nutrition: 160 Calories 10.7g Fat 2.7g Carbohydrates

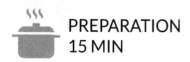

PREPARATION
15 MIN

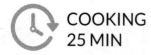

COOKING
25 MIN

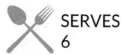

SERVES
6

25. BREAKFAST MUFFINS

INGREDIENTS

- 12 eggs
- 1/2 cup fresh spinach, shredded
- 1/4 tsp garlic powder
- 3/4 cup ham, diced and cooked
- 3 tbsp onion, chopped
- 1 cup cheddar cheese, shredded
- 1/4 cup mushrooms, chopped and sautéed
- 1/4 cup bell pepper, diced
- 1/4 tsp pepper
- 1/2 tsp salt

DIRECTIONS

Preheat the oven to 350 F.

Coat muffin tray with cooking spray and set aside.

In a large bowl, beat eggs. Add remaining ingredients to the bowl and mix well together.

Pour egg mixture into the prepared muffin tray.

Bake for 20-25 minutes.

Nutrition: 243 Calories 17g Fat 2.8g Carbohydrates

PREPARATION
5 MIN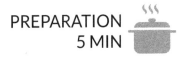

COOKING
10 MIN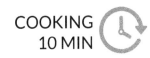

SERVES
4

26. CHOCÓ PEANUT BUTTER WAFFLE

INGREDIENTS

- 4 eggs, lightly beaten
- 2 1/2 tbsp unsweetened cocoa powder
- 1/4 cup Lakanto monk fruit
- 1/2 cup almond flour
- 1/3 cup unsweetened peanut butter
- 1/2 tsp baking powder, gluten-free

DIRECTIONS

Preheat the waffle maker.

Mix all ingredients.

Spray waffle maker with cooking spray.

Fill 1/4 cup of mixture onto the waffle maker and cook. Do with the remaining batter.

Nutrition: 271 Calories 20g Fat 6.5g Carbohydrates

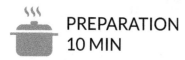

PREPARATION
10 MIN

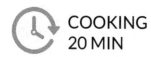

COOKING
20 MIN

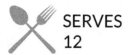

SERVES
12

27. CHEESE JALAPENO MUFFINS

INGREDIENTS

- 9 eggs
- 6 bacon slices
- 3/4 cup heavy cream
- 1 1/2 jalapeno pepper, sliced
- 8.5 oz cheddar cheese, shredded
- Pepper
- Salt

DIRECTIONS

Preheat the oven to 350 F.

Prep muffin tray with cooking spray and add cooked bacon slices to each muffin cup.

In a large bowl, whisk together eggs, cheese, cream, pepper, and salt.

Pour egg mixture into the prepared muffin tray.

Add sliced jalapeno into each muffin cup.

Bake for 15-20 minutes.

Nutrition: 228 Calories 18.4g Fat 1g Carbohydrates

PREPARATION
5 MIN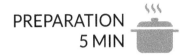

COOKING
15 MIN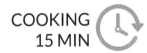

SERVES
6

28. SAUSAGE CHEESE CHAFFLES

INGREDIENTS

- ▸ 1/2 lb. Italian sausage
- ▸ 1/2 cup cheddar cheese, shredded
- ▸ 1/2 cup almond flour
- ▸ 1 egg, lightly beaten
- ▸ 2 tbsp parmesan cheese, grated

DIRECTIONS

Preheat waffle maker.

Combine all ingredients.

Spray waffle maker with cooking spray.

Pour 3 tbsp of mix in the waffle maker and cook. Repeat with the rest of the batter.

Nutrition: 234 Calories 19.4g Fat 2.6g Carbohydrates

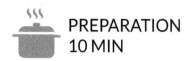

PREPARATION
10 MIN

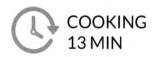

COOKING
13 MIN

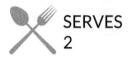

SERVES
2

29. TOMATO FRITTATA

INGREDIENTS

- 6 eggs
- 2/3 cup cherry tomatoes, halved
- 2/3 cup feta cheese, crumbled
- 1 small onion, sliced
- 1 tbsp chives, chopped
- 1 ½ tbsp basil, chopped
- 1 tbsp butter
- Pepper
- Salt

DIRECTIONS

Preheat the oven to 400 F.

Heat up butter in a pan over medium heat.

Sauté onion to the pan.

In a bowl, whisk eggs with chives, basil, pepper, and salt.

Once onions are done then add egg mixture and cook for 2-3 minutes.

Top with cheese and cherry tomatoes. Situate in oven and cook for 5-7 minutes.

Nutrition: 394 Calories 29g Fat 8g Carbohydrates

PREPARATION
5 MIN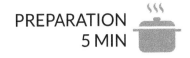

COOKING
15 MIN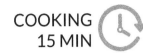

SERVES
2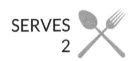

30. CHOCÓ CHIPS WAFFLE

INGREDIENTS

- 3 eggs
- 1/4 cup Swerve
- 1/2 cup butter
- 1/2 cup unsweetened chocolate chips
- 1/2 tsp vanilla

DIRECTIONS

Preheat the waffle maker.

Add chocolate chips and butter in microwave-safe bowl and microwave for 1 minute. Stir well.

In a bowl, whisk eggs with vanilla and Swerve until frothy.

Add melted butter and chocolate mixture in the egg mixture and stir well.

Spray waffle maker with cooking spray.

Pour 1/4 batter in the hot waffle maker and cook for 6-8 minutes or until golden brown. Repeat with the remaining batter.

Nutrition: 670 Calories 69g Fat 10g Carbohydrates

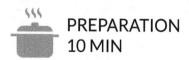
**PREPARATION
10 MIN**

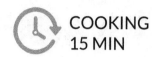
**COOKING
15 MIN**

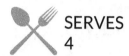
**SERVES
4**

31. CHEESE JALAPENO BREAD

INGREDIENTS

- 4 eggs
- 1/3 cup coconut flour
- 1/4 cup water
- 1/4 cup butter
- 1/4 tsp pepper
- 3 jalapeno chilies, chopped
- ¼ tsp onion powder
- 1/2 cup cheddar cheese, grated
- 1/4 cup parmesan cheese, grated
- 1/4 tsp baking powder, gluten-free

- 1/2 tsp garlic powder
- 1/2 tsp salt

DIRECTIONS

Preheat the oven to 400 F.

In a bowl, mix together eggs, pepper, salt, water, and butter.

Add baking powder, garlic powder, onion powder, and coconut flour and mix well.

Add jalapenos, cheddar cheese, and parmesan cheese. Mix well and season with pepper.

Line baking tray with parchment pepper.

Pour batter into a baking tray and spread evenly.

Bake for 15 minutes.

Nutrition: 249 Calories 22g Fat 2.7g Carbohydrates

PREPARATION
5 MIN

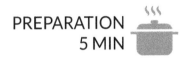

COOKING
10 MIN

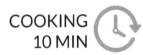

SERVES
2

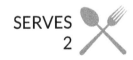

32. EASY HALLOUMI CHEESE CHAFFLES

INGREDIENTS

- 3 oz Halloumi cheese, cut into 1/2-inch thick slices

DIRECTIONS

Place cheese slice in the waffle maker and cook for 5-6 minutes or until golden brown. Repeat with the remaining cheese slice.

Nutrition: 155 Calories 12.7g Fat 1.1g Carbohydrates

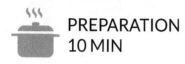

PREPARATION
10 MIN

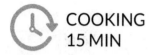

COOKING
15 MIN

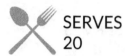

SERVES
20

33. PUMPKIN CINNAMON MUFFINS

INGREDIENTS

- ▸ 1/2 cup pumpkin puree
- ▸ 1/2 cup almond butter
- ▸ 1 tbsp cinnamon
- ▸ 1/2 cup coconut oil
- ▸ 1 tsp baking powder
- ▸ 2 scoops vanilla protein powder
- ▸ 1/2 cup almond flour

. . . .

DIRECTIONS

Preheat the oven to 350 F.

Grease muffin tray with cooking spray and set aside.

In a large bowl, mix together all dry ingredients.

Add wet ingredients into the dry ingredients and mix until well combined.

Pour batter into the prepared muffin tray and bake for 15 minutes.

Nutrition: 81 Calories 7.1g Fat 1.5g Carbohydrates

34. CHEESE CAULIFLOWER HASH BROWNS

PREPARATION
10 MIN
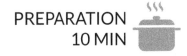

COOKING
15 MIN
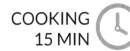

SERVES
6

INGREDIENTS

- 3 cups cauliflower, grated
- 3/4 cup cheddar cheese, shredded
- 1 egg, lightly beaten
- 1/2 tsp garlic powder
- 1/2 tsp cayenne pepper
- 1/4 tsp pepper
- 1/2 tsp salt

DIRECTIONS

Blend all ingredients into the bowl.

Grease baking tray with cooking spray and set aside.

Make six hash browns from cauliflower mixture and place on a prepared baking tray.

Bake at 400 F for 15 minutes.

Nutrition: 81 Calories 5g Fat 3.4g Carbohydrates

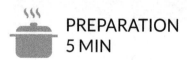

PREPARATION
5 MIN

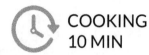

COOKING
10 MIN

SERVES
4

35. ALMOND FLOUR WAFFLE

INGREDIENTS

- ▶ 1 cup almond flour
- ▶ 4 eggs, lightly beaten
- ▶ 1/4 cup heavy cream
- ▶ Pinch of salt

. . . .

DIRECTIONS

Preheat the waffle maker.

Whisk all ingredients in a bowl.

Spray waffle maker with cooking spray.

Cook 1/4 batter in the waffle maker. Do it again with the rest.

Nutrition: 249 Calories 21g Fat 6g Carbohydrates

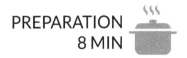

PREPARATION
8 MIN

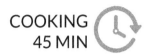

COOKING
45 MIN

36. TORTILLA BREAKFAST CASSEROLE

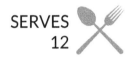

SERVES
12

INGREDIENTS

- 1 Pound Bacon, Cooked and Crumbled
- 1 Pound Pork Sausage. Cooked and Crumbled
- 1 Pound Package Diced Ham
- 10 8-inch Tortillas, Cut in half 8 Large Eggs
- 1 1/2 Cups Milk
- 1/2 Teaspoon Salt
- 1/2 Teaspoon Pepper
- 1/2 Teaspoon Garlic Powder
- 1/2 teaspoon Hot Sauce

- 2 Cups Shredded Cheddar Cheese
- 1 Cup Mozzarella or Monterrey Jack Cheese

DIRECTIONS

A 9x13-inch baking dish with 2 teaspoons of butter or sprinkle with nonstick spray oil.

Bake 1/3 layer of tortillas in the bottom of the pot and cover with baked bacon and 1/3 layer of cheese.

Place another third of the tortillas in the pan and cover with the cooked and chopped sausages and place another third of the cheese in layers.

Repeat with the last tortilla, ham and cheese 1/3.

In a big bowl, blend eggs, milk, salt, pepper, garlic powder, and hot sauce.

Pour the egg mixture evenly over the pot.

If desired, cover overnight and refrigerate or bake immediately.

When you are ready to bake, preheat the oven to 350 degrees.

Bake covered with foil for 45 minutes. Find and cook for another 20 minutes until the cheese is completely melted and cooked in a pan.

Nutrition: 447 calories 32.6 g fat 14.6 g carbohydrates

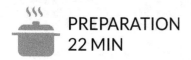

PREPARATION
22 MIN

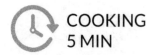

COOKING
5 MIN

SERVES
2

37. PECAN POPS

INGREDIENTS

- ▸ 4 large just-ripe bananas
- ▸ 2 tablespoons raw honey
- ▸ 4 Popsicle sticks
- ▸ 3A cup chopped pecans
- ▸ ½ cup almond butter

DIRECTIONS

Peel and cut one end from each banana, and insert a Popsicle stick into the cut end.

In a small bowl, scourge the almond butter and honey, and heat in the microwave for 10 to 15 seconds, or just until the mixture is slightly thinned. Put onto a sheet of wax paper and spread with a spatula.

On another piece of wax paper or foil, spread the chopped pecans — Line a small baking sheet or large plate with the third piece of wax paper or foil.

Roll each banana first in the honey mixture until well coated, then in the nuts until completely covered, pressing down gently, so the nuts adhere.

Place each finished banana onto the baking sheet. When all of the bananas have been coated, place the sheet in the freezer for at least 2 hours. For long-term storage, transfer the frozen bananas into a resealable plastic bag.

Nutrition: 14g Fat 7g Carbohydrates 19g Protein

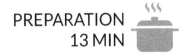

PREPARATION
13 MIN

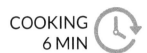

COOKING
6 MIN

38. GREEK BREAKFAST WRAPS

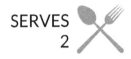

SERVES
2

INGREDIENTS

- ▸ 1 teaspoon olive oil
- ▸ ½ cup fresh baby spinach leaves
- ▸ 1 tablespoon fresh basil
- ▸ 4 egg whites, beaten
- ▸ ½ teaspoon salt
- ▸ ¼ teaspoon freshly ground black pepper
- ▸ ¼ cup crumbled low-fat feta cheese
- ▸ 2 (8-inch) whole-wheat tortillas

· ·

DIRECTIONS

Heat up olive oil on medium heat. Sauté spinach and basil to the pan for about 2 minutes.

Add the egg whites to the pan, season with the salt and pepper, and sauté, often stirring, for about 2 minutes more, or until the egg whites are firm.

Remove from the heat and sprinkle with the feta cheese.

Warm up tortillas in the microwave for 20 to 30 seconds. Divide the eggs between the tortillas and wrap up burrito-style.

Nutrition: 10.4g Fat 4.5g Carbohydrate 10.6g Protein

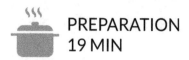

PREPARATION
19 MIN

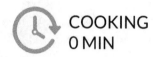

COOKING
0 MIN

SERVES
2

39. CURRIED CHICKEN BREAST WRAPS

INGREDIENTS

- 6 ounces cooked chicken breast
- 1 small Gala or Granny Smith apple
- 2 tablespoons plain low-fat yogurt
- 1 cup spring lettuce mix or baby lettuce
- 1 teaspoon Dijon mustard
- ½ teaspoon mild curry powder
- 2 (8-inch) whole-wheat tortillas

DIRECTIONS

Scourge chicken, yogurt, Dijon mustard, and curry powder; stir well to combine. Add the apple and stir until blended.

Portion the lettuce between the tortillas and top each with half of the chicken mixture. Roll up burrito-style and serve.

Nutrition: 5g fat 18g carbohydrates 28g protein

40. BAKED SALMON FILLETS WITH TOMATO AND MUSHROOMS

PREPARATION
8 MIN

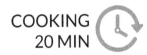

COOKING
20 MIN

SERVES
2

INGREDIENTS

- 2 (4-ounce) skin-on salmon fillets
- 2 teaspoons olive oil, divided
- ½ teaspoon salt
- ¼ teaspoon freshly ground black pepper
- ½ teaspoon chopped fresh dill
- ½ cup diced fresh tomato
- ½ cup sliced fresh mushrooms

DIRECTIONS

Prepare oven to 375 degrees F and line a baking sheet with aluminum foil.

You are using your fingers or a pastry brush, coat both sides of the fillets with ½ teaspoon of the olive oil each. Place the salmon skin-side down on the pan. Sprinkle salt and pepper equally all round.

In a small plate, mix the remaining 1 teaspoon olive oil, the tomato, mushrooms, and dill; stir well to combine. Spoon the mixture over the fillets.

Crease the sides and ends of the foil up to seal the fish, place the pan on the middle oven rack, and bake for about 20 minutes, or until the salmon flakes easily.

Nutrition: 12g Fat 21g Carbohydrate 25g Protein

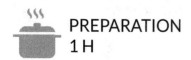

PREPARATION
1 H

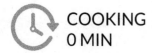

COOKING
0 MIN

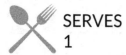

SERVES
1

41. CINNAMON AND SPICE OVERNIGHT OATS

INGREDIENTS

- 75g rolled oats
- 100ml milk
- 75g yogurt
- 1 tsp honey
- 1/2 tsp vanilla extract
- 1/8th tsp Schwartz ground cinnamon
- 20g raisins

DIRECTIONS

Incorporate all ingredients well. Chill overnight or at least one hour.

Remove from the fridge or heat it in the microwave immediately or slowly.

Nutrition: 15g Carbohydrates 26g Protein 34g Fat

PREPARATION
6 MIN

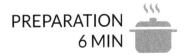

COOKING
50 MIN

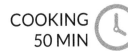

SERVES
6

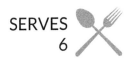

42. MEXICAN CASSEROLE

INGREDIENTS

- 1-pound lean ground beef
- 2 cups salsa
- 1 (16 ounces) can chili beans, drained
- 3 cups tortilla chips, crushed
- 2 cups sour cream
- 1 (2 ounces) can slice black olives, drained
- 1/2 cup chopped green onion
- 1/2 cup chopped fresh tomato
- 2 cups shredded Cheddar cheese

DIRECTIONS

Prep oven to 350 degrees Fahrenheit (175 degrees Celsius).

In a big wok over medium heat, cook the meat so that it is no longer pink. Add the sauce, reduce the heat and simmer for 20 minutes or until the liquid is absorbed. Add beans and heat.

Sprinkle a 9x13 baking dish with oil spray. Pour the chopped tortillas into the pan and then place the meat mixture on it. Pour sour cream over meat and sprinkle with olives, green onions, and tomatoes. Top with cheddar cheese.

Bake in preheated oven for 30 minutes or until hot and bubbly.

Nutrition: 43.7g fat 32.8g carbohydrates 31.7g protein

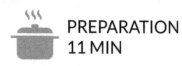
**PREPARATION
11 MIN**

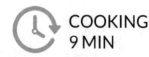
**COOKING
9 MIN**

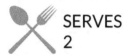
**SERVES
2**

43. MICROWAVED FISH AND ASPARAGUS WITH TARRAGON MUSTARD SAUCE

INGREDIENTS

- 12 ounces (340 g) fish fillets
- 10 asparagus spears
- 2 tablespoons (30 g) sour cream
- 1 tablespoon (15 g) mayonnaise
- ¼ teaspoon dried tarragon
- ½ teaspoon Dijon

DIRECTIONS

Draw the bottom of the asparagus spears and cut them naturally. Put the asparagus on a large glass plate, add 1 teaspoon (15 ml) of water and cover with a plate. Microwave for 3 minutes.

While the asparagus is in the microwave, mix sour, mayonnaise, tarragon and mustard together.

Remove the asparagus from the microwave oven, remove it from the pie plate and set aside. Drain the water from the runway. Put the fish fillet in it

Peel the pie plate and spread 2 tablespoons (30 ml) cream mixture on them and cover the pie again and place the fish in the microwave for 3 to 4 minutes. Open the oven, remove the plate from the top of the pie plate and place the asparagus on top of the fish. Cover the pie plate again and cook for another 1-2 minutes.

Remove the pie plate from the microwave oven and remove the plate. Put the fish and asparagus on a serving platter. Chop any boiled sauce on a plate over fish and asparagus. Melt each with reserved sauce and serve.

Nutrition: 4g carbohydrates 33 g protein 17g fat

PREPARATION 8 MIN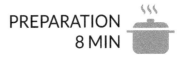

44. HEARTY HOT CEREAL WITH BERRIES

COOKING 20 MIN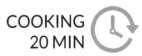

SERVES 4

INGREDIENTS

- ▶ 4 cups of water
- ▶ 2 tablespoons honey
- ▶ ½ teaspoon salt
- ▶ ½ cup fresh blueberries
- ▶ 2 cups whole rolled oats
- ▶ ½ cup fresh raspberries
- ▶ ½ cup chopped walnuts
- ▶ cup low-fat milk
- ▶ teaspoons flaxseed

. . . .

DIRECTIONS

In a saucepan, boil water at high heat and add the salt.

Stir in the oats, walnuts, and flaxseed, then reduce the heat to low and cover — Cook for 16 to 20 minutes, or until the oatmeal reaches the desired consistency.

Divide the oatmeal between 4 deep bowls and top each with 2 tablespoons of both blueberries and raspberries. Add ½ cup milk to each bowl and serve.

Nutrition: 15g Fat 17g Carbohydrates 19g Protein

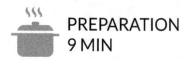

PREPARATION
9 MIN

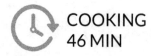

COOKING
46 MIN

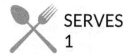

SERVES
1

45. PROTEIN SWEET POTATOES

INGREDIENTS

- 2 sweet potatoes
- 6 oz. plain Greek yogurt
- ½ tsp. salt
- 1/3 cup dried cranberries
- ¼ tsp. black pepper

DIRECTIONS

Set oven to 400 degrees and prick the sweet potatoes. Situate on a cooking plate and cook for 42 minutes.

Chop the potatoes in two and wrap the meat in a bowl and set aside skin.

Stir salt, pepper, yogurt, and cranberries.

Scoop the mix into the potato skins and serve.

Nutrition: 11g Fat 15g Carbohydrates 18g Protein

PREPARATION
7 MIN
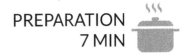

COOKING
19 MIN
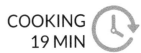

SERVES
2
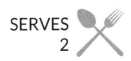

46. PENNE PASTA WITH VEGETABLES

INGREDIENTS

- ▶ 1 teaspoon salt, divided
- ▶ ¾ cup uncooked penne pasta
- ▶ 1 tablespoon olive oil
- ▶ 1 tablespoon chopped garlic
- ▶ 1 teaspoon chopped fresh oregano
- ▶ I cup sliced fresh mushrooms
- ▶ to cherry tomatoes, halved
- ▶ I cup fresh spinach leaves
- ▶ ½ teaspoon freshly ground black pepper
- ▶ 1 tablespoon shredded Parmesan cheese

DIRECTIONS

In a large saucepan, bring 1-quart water to a boil. Add 1/2 teaspoon of the salt and the penne, and cook according to package directions for 9 minutes. Drain but do not rinse the penne, reserving about VA cup pasta water.

Meanwhile, in a large skillet, heat the olive oil over medium-high heat. Add the garlic, oregano, and mushrooms, and sauté for 4 to 5 minutes, or until the mushrooms are golden.

Sauté tomatoes and spinach, season with the remaining ½ teaspoon salt and the black pepper for 4 minutes.

Cook drained pasta to the skillet, along with 2 to 3 tablespoons of the pasta water.

Constantly stirring, for 2 to 3 minutes.

Divide the pasta between two shallow bowls and sprinkle with the Parmesan cheese. Serve hot or at room temperature.

Nutrition: 12g Fat 9g Carbohydrates 19g Protein

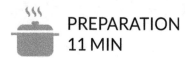

PREPARATION
11 MIN

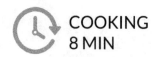

COOKING
8 MIN

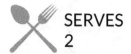

SERVES
2

47. SPINACH AND SWISS CHEESE OMELET

INGREDIENTS

- ▶ 1 teaspoon olive oil
- ▶ 6 large egg whites, beaten
- ▶ 1 cup fresh baby spinach leaves
- ▶ 2 (1-ounce) slices reduced-fat Swiss cheese
- ▶ ½ teaspoon salt
- ▶ ¼ teaspoon freshly ground black pepper

DIRECTIONS

In a small skillet, cook olive oil over medium-high heat. Sauté spinach, salt, and pepper for 3 minutes, stirring often.

Lay out spinach evenly at the bottom, and transfer egg whites over the top, leaning the pan to coat the spinach thoroughly.

Cook for 4 minutes, rarely pulling the edges of the eggs toward the center as you tilt the skillet to allow uncooked egg to spread to the sides of the pan.

Turnover eggs. Put the Swiss cheese cuts on one half of the omelet, and then turn it over to form a half-moon. Cook for 1 minute.

Nutrition: 8g Fat 12g Carbohydrates 18g Protein

PREPARATION
6 MIN
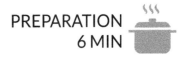

COOKING
17 MIN
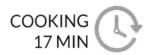

SERVES
2

48. BROILED HALIBUT WITH GARLIC SPINACH

INGREDIENTS

- 2 (4-ounce) halibut fillets, 1 inch thick
- ½ lemon (about 1 teaspoon juice)
- 1 teaspoon salt, divided
- ¼ teaspoon freshly ground black pepper
- ½ teaspoon cayenne pepper
- I teaspoon olive oil
- 2 cloves garlic
- ½ cup chopped red onion
- 2 cups fresh baby spinach leaves

DIRECTIONS

Prepare the broiler and position an oven rack 4 to 5 inches below the heat source. Line a baking sheet with aluminum foil.

Squeeze the lemon half over the fish fillets, then season each side with ½ teaspoon of the salt, pepper, and cayenne. Place the fish on the pan and broil for 8 minutes. Turn over the fish and cook for 7 minutes more.

Meanwhile, heat the olive oil in a small skillet over medium heat. Add the garlic and onion, and sauté for 2 minutes. Add the spinach and remaining ½ teaspoon salt, and sauté for 2 minutes more. Remove from the heat and cover to keep warm.

To serve, portion spinach between two plates and top with a fish fillet. Serve hot.

Nutrition: 22g Fat 17g Carbohydrates 19g Protein

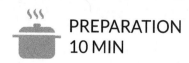
PREPARATION
10 MIN

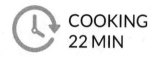
COOKING
22 MIN

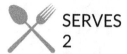
SERVES
2

49. QUINOA WITH CURRIED BLACK BEANS AND SWEET POTATOES

INGREDIENTS

- ½ cup quinoa
- ½ teaspoon dried rosemary
- 1 cup water
- 1 cup canned black beans
- ½ cup peeled and diced sweet
- 1 teaspoon mild curry powder potato
- 2 tablespoons chopped fresh parsley
- ½ teaspoon olive oil

DIRECTIONS

Wash quinoa in cold running water with a fine mesh sieve. Drain very well over paper towels and then pat dry.

In a small saucepan, toast the quinoa for 2 minutes over medium heat, shaking frequently. Add the water, increase the heat to high, and bring the water to a boil. Set in low, and cook for 15 minutes. Remove from the heat and cover to keep warm.

In a small bowl, toss the sweet potato with the olive oil and rosemary.

Transfer to a medium skillet over medium-high heat. Sauté, frequently stirring, for 7 minutes, or until well caramelized. Stir in the black beans and curry powder, reduce the heat to medium, and cook, frequently stirring, until the beans are heated through.

To serve, place ½ cup cooked quinoa on each plate and top with half of the bean mixture. Garnish with the parsley.

Nutrition: 22g Fat 17g Carbohydrates 19g Protein

50. QUINOA PILAF

PREPARATION
11 MIN
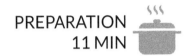

COOKING
20 MIN
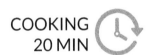

SERVES
4
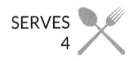

INGREDIENTS

- 2 tablespoons extra virgin olive oil
- 1/2 medium yellow onion
- 1/4 bell pepper
- 1 garlic clove
- 2 tablespoons pine nuts
- 1 cup uncooked quinoa
- 2 cups of water
- 2 tablespoons chopped fresh mint
- 2 tablespoons chopped fresh basil
- 1 tablespoon chopped fresh chives

- 1 small cucumber

DIRECTIONS

Rinse the box with instructions: check your quinoa box, if you recommend washing it, place the quinoa.in a large sieve and rinse it to remove water.

Onions, peppers, garlic, pine nuts: Heat 1 tbsp. Put the olive oil over medium-high heat in a pot of 1/1 to 2 quarts. Add and cook onions, rusty peppers, garlic and pine nuts, occasionally stirring until the onions are translucent but not browned.

Add quinoa: add and cook uncooked quinoa, occasionally stirring for a few minutes.

Add water, salt, stir: Add 2 glasses of water and a teaspoon of salt. Boil and decrease heat so that cheese and water shine while the pot is partially covered (enough for steam).

Cook for 20 minutes. Remove from heat and serve in a large bowl. Fill with a fork.

Add olive oil, mint, basil, onion, cucumber: add over low heat, add another tablespoon of olive oil. In chopped mint, mix basil, onion and cucumber. Add salt and pepper to taste.

Chill or cook at room temperature.

Nutrition: 22g Fat 17g Carbohydrates 19g Protein

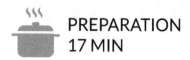

PREPARATION
17 MIN

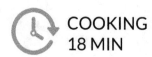

COOKING
18 MIN

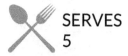

SERVES
5

51. CRISPY WAFFLES

INGREDIENTS

- ½ C. super fine almond flour
- ½ tsp. Swerve
- ¼ tsp. organic baking powder
- ¼ tsp. baking soda
- ¼ tsp. ground cinnamon
- 1/8 tsp. ground cloves
- 1/8 tsp. ground nutmeg
- ¼ tsp. salt
- 2 organic eggs
- 2 tbsp. butter, melted

- 1 tsp. organic vanilla extract

DIRECTIONS

In a bowl, add the flour, Swerve, baking powder, baking soda, spices and salt and mix well.

In a second bowl, add the egg yolks, butter and vanilla and beat until well combined.

In a third small bowl, add the egg whites and beat until soft peaks form.

Add the egg yolks mixture into flour mixture and mix until well combined.

Gently, fold in the beaten egg whites.

Place ¼ of the mixture into preheated waffle iron and cook for about 4-5 minutes or until golden brown.

Repeat with the remaining mixture.

Nutrition: 167 Calories 3.9g Carbohydrates 5.6g Protein

52. ANTI-INFLAMMATORY MUFFINS

PREPARATION
10 MIN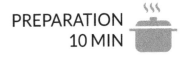

COOKING
23 MIN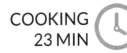

SERVES
6

INGREDIENTS

- 2 C. almond flour
- ½ C. powdered Swerve
- 3 scoops turmeric tonic
- 1½ tsp. organic baking powder
- 3 organic eggs
- 1 C. mayonnaise
- ½ tsp. organic vanilla extract

DIRECTIONS

Ready the oven to 350 degrees F. Line a 12 cups muffin tin with paper liners.

In a large bowl, add the flour, Swerve, turmeric tonic and baking powder and mix well.

Add the eggs, mayonnaise and vanilla extract and beat until well combined. Place the mixture into the prepared muffin cups evenly. Bake for about 20-23 minutes.

Pull out the muffin tin. Position onto the wire rack to cool for 8 minutes.

Carefully invert the muffins onto the wire rack to cool completely before serving.

Nutrition: 489 Calories 9.5g Carbohydrates 10.8g Protein

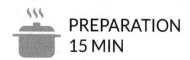
PREPARATION
15 MIN

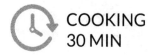
COOKING
30 MIN

SERVES
6

53. MINI CRUSTLESS QUICHES

INGREDIENTS

- 1 tsp. olive oil
- 1½ C. fresh mushrooms
- 1 scallion
- 1 tsp. garlic, mince
- 1 tsp. fresh rosemary, minced
- 1 (12.3-oz.) package lite firm silken tofu
- ¼ C. unsweetened almond milk
- 2 tbsp. Parmesan cheese
- 1 tbsp. arrowroot starch
- 1 tsp. butter, softened

- ¼ tsp. ground turmeric

DIRECTIONS

Set oven at 375 degrees F. Grease a 12 cups muffin tin.

In a nonstick skillet, heat the oil over medium heat and sauté the scallion and garlic for about 1 minute.

Add the mushrooms and sauté for about 5-7 minutes.

Stir in the rosemary and black pepper and remove from the heat

Set aside to cool slightly.

In a food processor, add the tofu and remaining ingredients and pulse until smooth.

Transfer the tofu mixture into a large bowl.

Fold in the mushroom mixture.

Place the mixture into the prepared muffin cups evenly.

Bake for about 20-22 minutes.

Remove the muffin pan from the oven and place onto a wire rack to cool for about 10 minutes.

Carefully, invert the muffins onto wire rack and serve warm.

Nutrition: 77 Calories 5.3g Carbohydrates 6.9g Protein

PREPARATION
10 MIN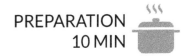

54. FRENCH BAKED EGGS

COOKING
12 MIN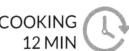

SERVES
4

INGREDIENTS

- ▶ 4 tbsp. half-and-half
- ▶ 4 organic eggs ½ oz. Gruyere cheese
- ▶ 4 tsp. fresh chives

DIRECTIONS

Ready the oven to 375 degrees F. Grease 4 ramekins.

In the bottom of each prepared ramekin, place 1 tbsp. of the heavy cream.

Carefully, crack 1 egg into each ramekin and sprinkle with the cheese, followed by salt, black pepper and chives.

Bake for about 8-12 minutes.

Nutrition: 97 Calories 1g Carbohydrates 7g Protein

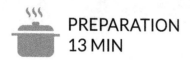

PREPARATION
13 MIN

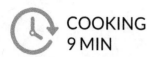

COOKING
9 MIN

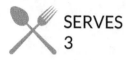

SERVES
3

55. ZINGY SCRAMBLE

INGREDIENTS

- ▶ 2 tbsp. unsalted butter
- ▶ 1 tomato
- ▶ 1 scallion
- ▶ 2 pickled jalapeños
- ▶ 6 organic eggs
- ▶ 3 oz. Colby jack cheese

· ·

DIRECTIONS

In a big frying pan, cook butter over medium-high heat and cook the tomato, scallion and jalapeños for about 3-4 minutes, stirring frequently.

Add the eggs and cook for about 2 minutes, stirring continuously.

Stir in the cheese, salt and black pepper and remove from the heat.

Nutrition: 235 Calories 2.7g Carbohydrates 13.2g Protein

PREPARATION
10 MIN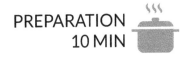

COOKING
0 MIN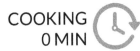

SERVES
1

56. NO-COOKING BREAKFAST BOWL

INGREDIENTS

- ▸ 2/3 C. frozen raspberries
- ▸ 1/3 C. frozen cauliflower rice
- ▸ 1 medium avocado
- ▸ 1 scoop unsweetened vanilla protein powder
- ▸ 1 tsp. beet powder
- ▸ ¼ C. unsweetened almond milk

DIRECTIONS

With high-speed blender, add all the ingredients and pulse until smooth.

Transfer into 2 serving bowls and serve with your favorite topping.

Nutrition: 125 Calories 8.9g Carbohydrates 14.3g Protein

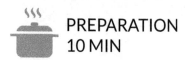

PREPARATION
10 MIN

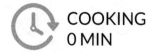

COOKING
0 MIN

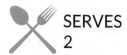

SERVES
2

57. SUPER FOOD SMOOTHIE BOWL

INGREDIENTS

- 2 C. fresh spinach
- 1 medium avocado
- 1 scoop unflavored collagen powder
- 1 scoop MCT oil powder
- ¼ C. Erythritol
- 2 tbsp. fresh lemon juice
- 1 C. unsweetened almond milk
- ¼ C. Ice cubes

DIRECTIONS

Using high-speed blender, add all the ingredients and pulse until smooth.

Transfer into 2 serving bowls and serve with your favorite topping.

Nutrition: 304 Calories 12g Carbohydrates 17g Protein

PREPARATION
15 MIN
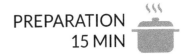

COOKING
35 MIN
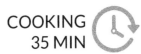

SERVES
5

58. NUTTY TEXTURED PORRIDGE

INGREDIENTS

- ▸ ½ C. pecans
- ▸ ½ C. walnuts
- ▸ ¼ C. sunflower seeds
- ▸ ¼ C. chia seeds
- ▸ ¼ C. unsweetened coconut flakes
- ▸ 4 C. unsweetened almond milk
- ▸ ½ tsp. ground cinnamon
- ▸ ¼ tsp. ground ginger
- ▸ 1 tsp. stevia powder
- ▸ 1 tbsp. butter

DIRECTIONS

In a food processor, place the pecans, walnuts and sunflower seeds and pulse until a crumbly mixture is formed.

In a large pan, add the nuts mixture, chia seeds, coconut flakes, almond milk, spices and stevia powder over medium heat and bring to a gentle simmer, stirring frequently.

Select heat to low and simmer for about 20-30 minutes, stirring frequently.

Remove from the heat and serve hot with the topping of butter.

Nutrition: 269 Calories 8.6g Carbohydrates 7g Protein

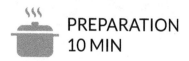

PREPARATION
10 MIN

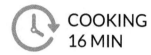

COOKING
16 MIN

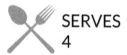

SERVES
4

59. CHEESY CAULIFLOWER CROQUETTES

INGREDIENTS

- 2 c. cauliflower florets
- 2 tsps. minced garlic
- ½ c. chopped onion
- ¾ tsp. mustard
- ½ tsp. salt
- ½ tsp. pepper
- 2 tbsps. butter
- ¾ c. grated cheddar cheese

DIRECTIONS

Place butter in a microwave-safe bowl then melts the butter. Let it cool. Place cauliflower florets in a food processor then process until smooth and becoming crumbles. Transfer the cauliflower crumbles to a bowl then add chopped onion and cheese.

Season with minced garlic, mustard, salt, and pepper then pour melted butter over the mixture. Shape the cauliflower mixture into medium balls then arrange in the Air Fryer.

Prepare the Air Fryer to 400°F (204°C) and cook the cauliflower croquettes for 14 minutes.

To achieve a more golden-brown color, cook the cauliflower croquettes for another 2 minutes.

Serve and enjoy with homemade tomato sauce.

Nutrition: 160 Calories 13g Fat: 6g Protein

60. SPINACH IN CHEESE ENVELOPES

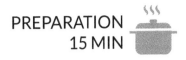
PREPARATION
15 MIN

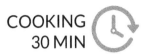
COOKING
30 MIN

SERVES
8

INGREDIENTS

- 3 c. cream cheese
- 1½ c. coconut flour
- 3 egg yolks
- 2 eggs
- ½ c. cheddar cheese
- 2 c. steamed spinach
- ¼ tsp. salt
- ½ tsp. pepper
- ¼ c. chopped onion

DIRECTIONS

Place cream cheese in a mixing bowl then whisks until soft and fluffy. Add egg yolks to the mixing bowl then continue whisking until incorporated.

Stir in coconut flour to the cheese mixture then mix until becoming a soft dough. Place the dough on a flat surface then roll until thin. Cut the thin dough into 8 squares then keep. Crash the eggs then place in a bowl. Season with salt, pepper, and grated cheese then mix well. Add chopped spinach and onion to the egg mixture then stir until combined.

Put spinach filling on a square dough then fold until becoming an envelope. Repeat with the remaining spinach filling and dough. Glue with water. Preheat an Air Fryer to 425°F (218°C). Arrange the spinach envelopes in the Air Fryer then cook for 12 minutes or until lightly golden brown.

Remove from the Air Fryer then serve warm. Enjoy!

Nutrition: 365 Calories 34g Fat 10g Protein

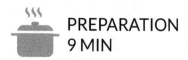 **PREPARATION**
9 MIN

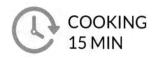 **COOKING**
15 MIN

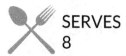 **SERVES**
8

61. CHEESY MUSHROOM SLICES

INGREDIENTS

- ► 2 c. chopped mushrooms
- ► 2 eggs
- ► ¾ c. almond flour
- ► ½ c. grated cheddar cheese
- ► 2 tbsps. butter
- ► ½ tsp. pepper
- ► ¼ tsp. salt

DIRECTIONS

Place butter in a microwave-safe bowl then melts the butter.

Place chopped mushrooms in a food processor then add eggs, almond flour, and cheddar cheese.

Season with salt and pepper then pour melted butter into the food processor. Process until mixed. Transfer to a silicone loaf pan then spread evenly.

Preheat an Air Fryer to 375°F (191°C).

Place the loaf pan on the Air Fryer's rack then cook for 15 minutes. Once it is done, remove from the Air Fryer then let it cool.

Cut the mushroom loaf into slices then serve.

Nutrition: 365 Calories 34g Fat 10g Protein

PREPARATION
9 MIN
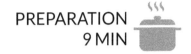

COOKING
11 MIN
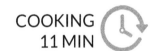

SERVES
4
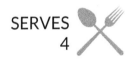

62. VEGGIE FRIES

INGREDIENTS

- Medium organic asparagus spears – 10
- Mayonnaise, full-fat – 3 tablespoons
- Organic roasted red pepper, chopped – 1 tablespoon
- Almond flour – ¼ cup
- Garlic powder – ½ teaspoon
- Smoked paprika – ½ teaspoon
- Chopped parsley – 2 tablespoons
- Parmesan cheese, grated and full-fat – ½ cup

- Organic eggs, beaten – 2

DIRECTIONS

Set oven to 425 degrees F and preheat. Meanwhile, place cheese in a food processor, add garlic and parsley and pulse for 1 minute until fine mixture comes together.

Add almond flour, pulse for 30 seconds until just mixed, then tip the mixture into a bowl and season with paprika. Beat eggs into a shallow dish.

Working on one asparagus spear at a time, first dip into the egg mixture, then coat with parmesan mixture and place it on a baking sheet.

Dip and coat more asparagus in the same manner, then arrange them on a baking sheet, 1-inch apart, and bake in the oven

for 10 minutes or until asparagus is tender and nicely golden brown.

Meanwhile, place mayonnaise in a bowl, add red pepper and whisk until combined and chill the dip into the refrigerator until required. Serve asparagus with prepared dip.

Nutrition: 453 Calories 33g Fat 19g Protein

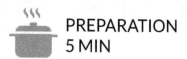

PREPARATION
5 MIN

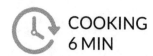

COOKING
6 MIN

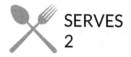

SERVES
2

63. ZUCCHINI NOODLES

INGREDIENTS

- Medium zucchini, spiralized into noodles – 2
- Butter, unsalted – 2 tablespoons
- Minced garlic – 1 ½ tablespoon
- Parmesan cheese, grated – 3/4 cup
- Sea salt – ½ teaspoon
- Ground black pepper – ¼ teaspoon
- Red chili flakes – ¼ teaspoon

DIRECTIONS

Switch on the instant pot, add butter, press the 'sauté/simmer' button, wait until the butter melts, and add garlic and cook for 1 minute or until fragrant.

Add zucchini noodles, toss until coated, cook for 5 minutes or until tender and season with salt and black pepper.

Press the 'keep warm' button, then transfer to noodles to a dish, top with cheese and sprinkle with red chili flakes.

Serve straight away.

Nutrition: 298 Calories 26g Fat 5g Protein

PREPARATION
10 MIN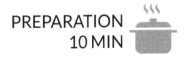

64. CAULIFLOWER SOUFFLE

COOKING
12 MIN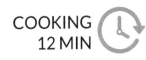

SERVES
6

INGREDIENTS

- Big head of Cauliflower– 1
- Eggs – 2
- Heavy Cream – 2 tablespoons
- Cream Cheese – 2 ounces
- Sour Cream – 1/2 cup
- Asiago cheese – 1/2 cup
- Sharp Cheddar Cheese, grated – 1 cup
- Chives – ¼ cup
- Butter, unsalted – 2 tablespoons
- slices of bacon, sugar-free, cooked, crumbled – 6
- Water – 1 cup

DIRECTIONS

Crack eggs in a food processor, add heavy cream, sour cream, cream cheese, and cheeses and pulse until smooth. Add cauliflower florets, pulse for 2 seconds or until folded and chunky, then add butter and chives and pulse for another 2 seconds.

Switch on the instant pot, pour in water, and insert a trivet stand. Pour the cauliflower mixture in a greased round casserole dish that fits into the instant pot, smooth the top and place the dish on the trivet stand.

Shut the instant pot with its lid in the sealed position, then press the 'manual' button, press '+/-' to set the cooking time to 12 minutes and cook at high-pressure setting; when the pressure builds in the pot, the cooking timer will start.

When the instant pot buzzes, press the 'keep warm' button, release pressure naturally for 10 minutes, then do a quick pressure release and open the lid. Take out the casserole dish, top with bacon, and serve.

Nutrition: 342 Calories 28g Fat 17g Protein

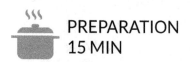

PREPARATION
15 MIN

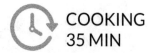

COOKING
35 MIN

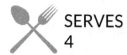

SERVES
4

65. SCRUMPTIOUS CAULIFLOWER CASSEROLE

INGREDIENTS

- 1 large head cauliflower
- 2 tbsp. butter
- 2 oz. cream cheese
- 1¼ C. sharp cheddar cheese
- 1 C. heavy cream
- ¼ C. scallion

DIRECTIONS

Preheat the oven to 350 0 F.

In a huge pan of boiling water, mix the cauliflower florets and cook for about 2 minutes.

Drain cauliflower and keep aside.

For cheese sauce: in a medium pan, add butter over medium-low heat and cook until just melted.

Add cream cheese, 1 C. of cheddar cheese, heavy cream, salt and black pepper and cook until melted and smooth, stirring continuously.

Pull away from heat and keep aside to cool slightly.

In a baking dish, place cauliflower florets, cheese sauce, and 3 tbsp. of scallion and stir to combine well.

Sprinkle with remaining cheddar cheese and scallion.

Bake for about 30 minutes.

Remove the casserole dish from oven and set aside for about 5-10 minutes before serving.

Cut into 4 equal-sized portions and serve.

Nutrition: 365 Calories 5.6g Carbohydrates 12g Protein

CHAPTER 4. LUNCH RECIPES

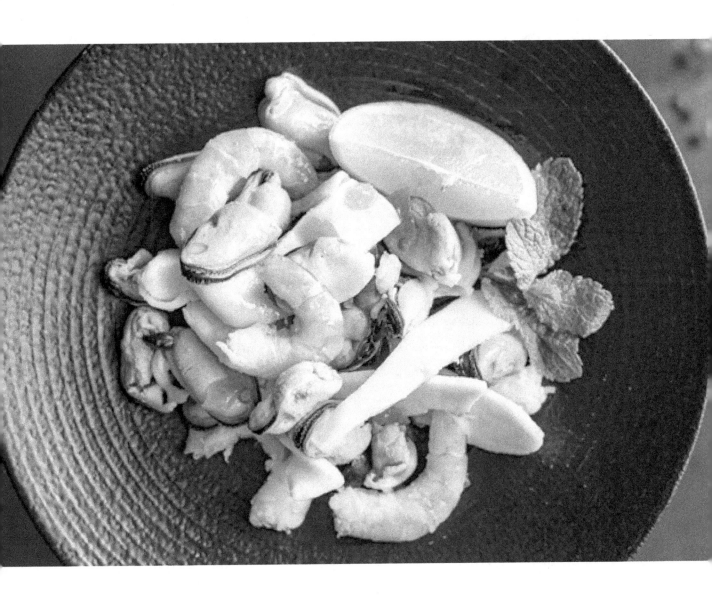

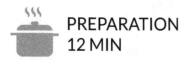

PREPARATION
12 MIN

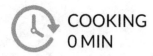

COOKING
0 MIN

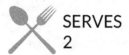

SERVES
2

66. LOW-CARB SMOKED SALMON LUNCH BOWL

INGREDIENTS

- 12-ounce smoked salmon
- 4 tbsp mayonnaise
- 2-ounce spinach
- 1 tbsp. olive oil
- 2 medium lime

DIRECTIONS

Situate mayonnaise, salmon, spinach on a plate.

Drizzle olive oil over the spinach.

Serve with lime wedges and season.

Nutrition: 460 calories 3g carbohydrates 36g fats

67. EASY ONE-PAN GROUND BEEF AND GREEN BEANS

PREPARATION
13 MIN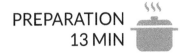

COOKING
6 MIN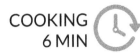

SERVES
2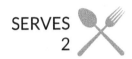

INGREDIENTS

- Ten ounces (80/20) ground beef
- Nine ounces green beans
- Pepper and salt, to taste
- 2 tbsp. sour cream
- 3½ oz butter

DIRECTIONS

Rinse green beans, then trim the ends off each side.

Place half of the butter to a pan (that can fit the ground green beans and beef) over high heat.

Once hot, stir in the ground beef and season. Cook the beef until it's almost done.

Set heat on the pan to medium. Cook rest of butter and green beans to the pan for five minutes. Stir the ground beef and green beans rarely.

Season the green beans, with the pan drippings.

Nutrition: 787.5 Calories 71.75g Fats 27.5g Protein.

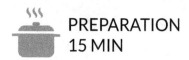
PREPARATION
15 MIN

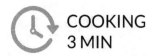
COOKING
3 MIN

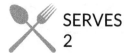
SERVES
2

68. EASY SPINACH AND BACON SALAD

INGREDIENTS

- ► Eight ounces spinach
- ► Four large hard-boiled eggs
- ► 6 ounces bacon
- ► One/Two medium red onion, thinly sliced
- ► One/Two cup mayonnaise
- ► Pepper and salt, to taste

DIRECTIONS

Fry bacon until it is done and crispy. Cut into pieces once cooked and set aside.

Chop the hard-boiled eggs and, if necessary, rinse the spinach.

Mix lettuce, mayonnaise, and remaining bacon fat into a huge cup, season.

Throw red onion, sliced eggs, and bacon into the salad. Serve.

Nutrition: 46g Fats 508 Calories 20g Protein.

PREPARATION
12 MIN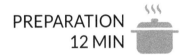

COOKING
0 MIN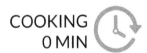

SERVES
2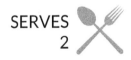

69. EASY KETO ITALIAN PLATE

INGREDIENTS

- ▶ Seven ounces fresh mozzarella cheese
- ▶ Seven ounces prosciutto
- ▶ Two medium tomatoes
- ▶ Four tablespoons olive oil
- ▶ Ten whole green olives
- ▶ Pepper and salt, to taste

DIRECTIONS

Situate tomato, olives, mozzarella, and prosciutto on a plate.

Season the tomato and cheese well. Serve with olive oil, either for dipping or drizzling.

Nutrition: 780.98 Calories 60.74g Fats 50.87g Protein.

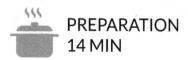

PREPARATION
14 MIN

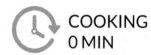

COOKING
0 MIN

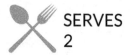

SERVES
2

70. FRESH BROCCOLI AND DILL KETO SALAD

INGREDIENTS

- 16 ounces broccoli
- One/Two cup mayonnaise
- 3/4 cup chopped fresh dill
- Salt and pepper, to taste

DIRECTIONS

Slice broccoli into tiny pieces. Chop stems into even smaller pieces.

Carry a saucepan of salted water to boil. Add the broccoli to the pot and boil for 3-5 minutes until slightly softened. The broccoli should still be bright green and crisp. Drain the broccoli and set aside to cool.

Once broccoli is cooled, add the remaining ingredients and stir together to combine. Season with pepper and salt, serve afterward.

Nutrition: 303.33 Calories 28.1g Fats 4.03g Protein

71. KETO SMOKED SALMON FILLED AVOCADOS

PREPARATION 13 MIN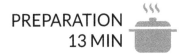

COOKING 5 MIN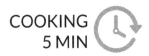

SERVES 2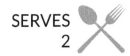

INGREDIENTS

- One medium avocado
- Three ounces smoked salmon
- Four tablespoons sour cream
- One tablespoon lemon juice
- Pepper and salt, to taste

DIRECTIONS

Cut the avocado(s) into two and discard the pit.

Place the same amounts of sour cream in the hollow parts of the avocado. Include smoked salmon on top.

Season with pepper and salt, squeeze lemon juice over the top.

Nutrition: 517 Calories 42.6g Fats 20.6g Protein.

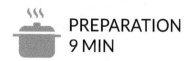

PREPARATION
9 MIN

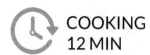

COOKING
12 MIN

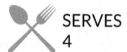

SERVES
4

72. LOW-CARB BROCCOLI LEMON PARMESAN SOUP

INGREDIENTS

- Three cups water
- One cup unsweetened almond milk
- Thirty-two ounces broccoli florets
- One cup heavy whipping cream
- 3/4 cup shredded Parmesan cheese
- Salt and pepper, to taste
- Two tablespoons lemon juice

DIRECTIONS

In a dish, add the broccoli and water and cook over medium-high heat until broccoli is tender.

Take from the pot One cup of the cooking liquid, and remove the rest.

In a blender, add half the broccoli, reserved cooking oil, unsweetened almond milk, heavy cream, and salt and pepper. Mix well until smooth.

In the pot, add the blended ingredients to the remaining broccoli, and stir with Parmesan cheese and lemon juice. Continue cooking until heated through.

Where needed, taste, and season with extra salt and pepper. Serve with Parmesan cheese sprinkled over the top.

Nutrition: 371 Calories 28.38g Fats 14.63g Protein.

PREPARATION
17 MIN

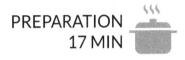

COOKING
6 MIN

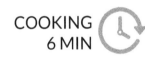

SERVES
3

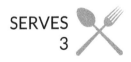

73. PROSCIUTTO AND MOZZARELLA BOMB

INGREDIENTS

- ▶ Four ounces sliced prosciutto
- ▶ Eight ounces fresh mozzarella ball
- ▶ Olive oil, for frying

DIRECTIONS

Layer half of the prosciutto slices vertically. Lay the remaining slices horizontally across the first set of slices.

Place your mozzarella ball, upside down, onto the crisscrossed prosciutto slices.

Firmly, but very carefully, wrap the mozzarella ball with the prosciutto slices.

If making ahead, wrap the balls in cling film and refrigerate.

Heat the olive oil in a skillet, afterward crisp the prosciutto on all sides, then serve

Nutrition: 253 Calories 19.35g Fats 18g Protein.

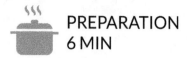

PREPARATION
6 MIN

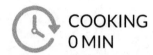

COOKING
0 MIN

SERVES
3

74. SUMMER TUNA AVOCADO SALAD

INGREDIENTS

- One can tuna flakes or chunks (approx. 120g)
- One medium avocado, chopped
- One medium English cucumber, chopped
- ¼ cup cilantro, chopped
- One tbsp lemon juice
- One tbsp olive oil
- Pepper and salt, to taste

DIRECTIONS

Put the first 4 ingredients into a salad bowl.

Sprinkle with the lemon and olive oil

Nutrition: 303 Calories 22.6g Fats 16.7g Protein.

75. MUSHROOMS & GOAT CHEESE SALAD

PREPARATION
12 MIN
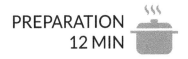

COOKING
8 MIN
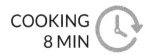

SERVES
2

INGREDIENTS

- One tablespoon butter
- Two ounces cremini mushrooms, sliced
- Pepper and salt, to taste
- Four ounces spring mix
- One-ounce cooked bacon, crumbled
- One-ounce goat cheese, crumbled
- One tablespoon olive oil
- One tablespoon balsamic vinegar

DIRECTIONS

Heat the saucepan with the butter in it over medium.

Sautee until the mushrooms are soft and brown. Season with pepper and salt to taste.

Place the salad greens in a bowl. Top with goat cheese and crumbled bacon.

Mix these in the salad once the mushrooms are done.

Whisk the olive oil in a small bowl, and balsamic vinegar together. Put the salad on top and serve.

Nutrition: 243 calories 21g fat 1g fiber

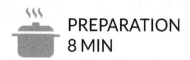

PREPARATION
8 MIN

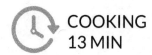

COOKING
13 MIN

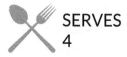

SERVES
4

76. KETO BACON SUSHI

INGREDIENTS

- Six slices bacon, halved
- One avocado, sliced
- Two Persian cucumbers, thinly sliced
- Two medium carrots, thinly sliced
- Four oz. cream cheese, softened

DIRECTIONS

Preheat oven to 400F Line a baking sheet with aluminum foil and fit it with a cooling rack. Place bacon halves in an even layer and bake until slightly fresh but still pliable, 11 to 13 minutes.

Meanwhile, slice cucumbers, avocado, and carrots into sections roughly the width of the bacon.

When bacon is cold enough to touch, spread an even layer of cream cheese on both slices. Divide vegetables evenly between the bacon and place on one end. Roll up vegetables tightly.

Garnish and serve.

Nutrition: 11g carbohydrates 28g protein 30g fat

PREPARATION
7 MIN

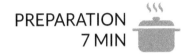

COOKING
39 MIN

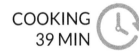

SERVES
4

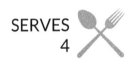

77. KETO PAPRIKA CHICKEN

INGREDIENTS

- Four Boneless, Skinless Chicken Breasts
- Three Tbsp. Olive Oil
- Two Tbsp. Spanish Smoked Paprika
- One Tbsp. Maple Syrup
- Two Tbsp. Lemon Juice (One Lemon)
- Salt and Pepper
- Two tsp. Minced Garlic

DIRECTIONS

Oven preheats to 350F.

Prepare chicken, cut into chunks and season with salt and pepper. Then, combine all other ingredients to prepare the sauce.

Add 1/3 of sauce to the bottom of a casserole dish and top with the chicken.

Spread the rest of the sauce thoroughly overall chicken parts then place in the oven for 35 minutes.

Broil the chicken for an additional 4-5 minutes to finish off.

Nutrition: 274 Calories 13.6g Fats 36.4g Protein

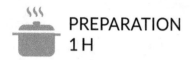
PREPARATION
1 H

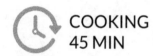
COOKING
45 MIN

SERVES
6

78. PERFECT SUNDAY ROAST

INGREDIENTS

- five lbs. beef rib roast
- two tsp. salt
- one tsp. pepper
- one tsp. garlic powder

DIRECTIONS

Let the roast stand for 60 minutes to room temperature.

Oven preheats to 375F. Combine all the spices.

On a roasting rack, place the rib roast, or inside a saucepan. Apply spices on the roast.

Roast in the oven for 1 hour. Switch off the oven, and do NOT open the door. Allow roast rest in the oven for 3 hours.

Turn oven back on to 375F for 30 - 45 minutes before serving.

Take it off the oven and let rest for ten minutes before cutting.

Nutrition: 1098 Calories 78g Protein 2594mg Cholesterol

79. BACON ROASTED CHICKEN WITH PAN GRAVY

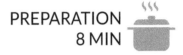

PREPARATION
8 MIN

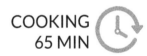

COOKING
65 MIN

SERVES
8

INGREDIENTS

▸ Three lbs. Whole Chicken, gutted
▸ Four sprigs Fresh Thyme
▸ One medium Lemon
▸ Ten strips bacon
▸ Salt and Pepper to Taste
▸ One tbsp. Grain Mustard

DIRECTIONS

Oven preheats to 500F. Season with salt and pepper, then lemon stuff, and thyme. Cover bacon with salt and pepper over bird skin, and season bacon.

Place the bird in a roasting saucepan and place it in the oven for 15 minutes. Reduce the temperature to 350F and bake for 40-50 minutes.

Remove birds and put them in foil. Drizzle the juices into a pan and bring to a boil.

Add mustard, stir in, and slightly reduce to pan liquids. Then, use an immersion blender to blend sauce into the pan.

Serve with gravy on chicken.

Nutrition: 376 Calories 29.8g Fats 24.5g Protein.

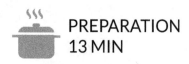

PREPARATION
13 MIN

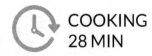

COOKING
28 MIN

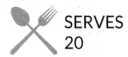

SERVES
20

80. CRISPY SKIN SLOW ROASTED PORK SHOULDER

INGREDIENTS

- Eight lbs. Pork Shoulder
- Three One/Two tbsp. Salt
- Two tsp. Oregano
- One tsp. Black Pepper
- One tsp. Garlic Powder
- One tsp. Onion Powder

. . . .

DIRECTIONS

Rinse the pork and leave it out for a few hours to reach room temperature. Rub salt and spices over the entire pork shoulder and preheat oven to 250F

Place on a wire rack that sits over a foil-covered baking sheet. Bake for eight to ten hours (more or less depending on size), or until around 190F internal temperature.

Remove meat from the frying pan and cover with foil. Set it to rest for fifteen min. Heat oven to 500F meanwhile.

Remove foil and roast pork over at 500F for a minimum of 20 minutes, rotating every five min.

Let the pork rest for fifteen to twenty minutes before they are cut and served.

Nutrition: 461 Calories 36.7g Fats 30.3g Protein

81. COLE SLAW KETO WRAP

PREPARATION
15 MIN
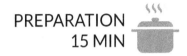

COOKING
0 MIN
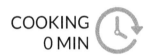

SERVES
2

INGREDIENTS

- Red Cabbage (3 cups sliced thin)
- Green Onions (0.5 cups, diced)
- Mayo (0.75 cups)
- Apple Cider Vinegar (2 teaspoons)
- Salt (0.25 teaspoon)
- Collard Green (16 pieces, stems removed)
- Ground Meat of choice (1 pound, cooked & chilled)
- Alfalfa Sprouts (0.33 cup)
- Toothpicks (to hold wraps together)

. . . .

DIRECTIONS

Mix slaw items with a spoon in a large-sized bowl until everything is well-coated.

Place a collard green on a plate and scoop a tablespoon or two of coleslaw on the edge of the leaf. Top it with a scoop of meat and sprouts.

Roll and tuck the sides to keep the filling from spilling.

Once you assemble the wrap, put in your toothpicks in a way that holds the wrap together until you are ready to beat it. Just repeat this with the leftover leaves.

Nutrition: 409 Calories 2g Fiber 2g Protein

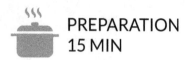

PREPARATION
15 MIN

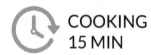

COOKING
15 MIN

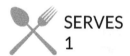

SERVES
1

82. KETO CHICKEN CLUB LETTUCE WRAP

INGREDIENTS

- ▸ 1 head of iceberg lettuce with the core and outer leaves removed
- ▸ 1 tbsp. of mayonnaise
- ▸ 6 slices or organic chicken or turkey breast
- ▸ Bacon (2 cooked strips, halved)
- ▸ Tomato (just 2 slices)

DIRECTIONS

Line your working surface with a large slice of parchment paper.

Layer 6-8 large leaves of lettuce in the center of the paper to make a base of around 9-10 inches.

Spread the mayo in the center and lay with chicken or turkey, bacon, and tomato.

Starting with the end closest to you, roll the wrap like a jelly roll with the parchment paper as your guide. Keep it tight and halfway through, roll tuck in the ends of the wrap.

When it is completely wrapped, roll the rest of the parchment paper around it, and use a knife to cut it in half.

Nutrition: 2g Fiber 28g Protein 837 Calories

PREPARATION
10 MIN

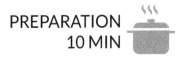

COOKING
0 MIN

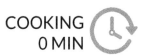

SERVES
4-6

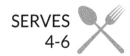

83. KETO BROCCOLI SALAD

INGREDIENTS

- **For your salad**
- Broccoli (2 medium-sized heads, florets chunked)
- Red Cabbage (2 cups shredded well)
- Sliced Almonds (0.5 cups, roasted)
- Green Onions (1 stalk, sliced)
- Raisins (0.5 cups)
- For your orange almond dressing
- Orange Juice (0.33 cup)
- Almond Butter (0.25 cup)

- Coconut Aminos (2 tablespoons)
- Shallot (1; small-sized, chopped finely)
- Salt (a half-teaspoon)

. . . .

DIRECTIONS

Use a food processor to pulse together salt, shallot, amino, nut butter, and OJ. Make sure it is perfectly smooth.

Use a medium-sized bowl to combine other ingredients. Toss it with dressing and serve.

Nutrition: 94g Fat 22g Protein 1022 Calories

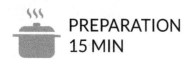

PREPARATION
15 MIN

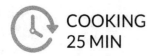

COOKING
25 MIN

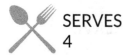

SERVES
4

84. KETO SHEET PAN CHICKEN AND RAINBOW VEGGIES

INGREDIENTS

- Nonstick spray
- Chicken Breasts (1 pound, boneless & skinless)
- Sesame Oil (1 tablespoon)
- Soy Sauce (2 tablespoons)
- Honey (2 tablespoons)
- Red Pepper (2; medium-sized, sliced)
- Yellow Pepper (2; medium-sized, sliced)
- Carrots (3; medium-sized, sliced)
- Broccoli (half-a-head cut up)

- 2 Red Onions (medium-size and sliced)
- EVOO (2 tablespoons)
- Pepper & salt (to taste)
- Parsley (0.25 cup, fresh herb, chopped)

DIRECTIONS

Cover baking sheet with cooking spray and bring the oven to a temperature of 400-degrees

Put the chicken in the middle of the sheet. Separately, combine the oil and the soy sauce. Brush the mix over the chicken.

Like the image above shows, separate your veggies across the plate. Sprinkle with oil and then toss them gently to ensure they are coated. Finally, spice up with pepper & salt.

Set tray into the oven and cook for around 25 minutes until all is tender and done throughout.

After taking out of the oven, garnish using parsley. Divide everything between those prep containers paired with your favorite greens.

Nutrition: 30g Fat 30g Protein 437 Calories

85. SKINNY BANG-BANG ZUCCHINI NOODLES

PREPARATION 15 MIN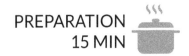

COOKING 15 MIN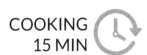

SERVES 4

INGREDIENTS

- **For the noodles**
- 4 medium zucchinis spiraled
- 1 tbsp. olive oil
- **For the sauce**
- Plain Greek Yogurt (0.25 cup + 2 tablespoons)
- Mayo (0.25 cup + 2 tablespoons)
- Thai Sweet Chili Sauce (0.25 cup + 2 tablespoons)
- Honey (1.5 teaspoons)

- Sriracha (1.5 teaspoons)
- Lime Juice (2 teaspoons)

DIRECTIONS

If you are using any meats for this dish such as chicken or shrimp, cook them first then set aside.

Pour the oil into a large-sized skillet at medium temperature.

After the oil heats through, stir in the spiraled zucchini noodles.

Cook the "noodles" until tender yet still crispy.

Remove from the heat, drain, and set at rest for at least 10 minutes.

Combine sauce items together into a large-sized both until perfectly smooth.

Divide into 4 small containers. Mix your noodles with any meats you cooked and add to meal prep containers.

Nutrition: 1g Fat 9g Protein 161 Calories

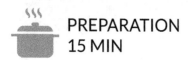

PREPARATION
15 MIN

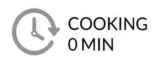

COOKING
0 MIN

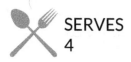

SERVES
4

86. KETO CAESAR SALAD

INGREDIENTS

- Mayonnaise (1.5 cups)
- Apple Cider Vinegar / ACV (3 tablespoons)
- Dijon Mustard (1 teaspoon)
- Anchovy Filets (4)
- Romaine Heart Leaves (24 of them)
- Pork Rinds (4 ounces, chopped)
- Parmesan (for garnish)

DIRECTIONS

Place the mayo with ACV, mustard, and anchovies into a blender and process until smooth and dressing like.

Prepare romaine leaves and pour out dressing across them evenly. Top with pork rinds and enjoy.

Nutrition: 3g Fiber 86g Fat 993 Calories

87. KETO BUFFALO CHICKEN EMPANADAS

PREPARATION
20 MIN
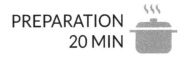

COOKING
30 MIN
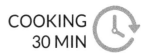

SERVES
6

INGREDIENTS

- **For the empanada dough**
- 1 ½ cups of mozzarella cheese
- 3 oz of cream cheese
- 1 whisked egg
- 2 cups of almond flour
- **For the buffalo chicken filling**
- 2 cups of cooked shredded chicken
- Butter (2 tablespoons, melted)
- Hot Sauce (0.33 cup)

DIRECTIONS

Bring the oven to a temperature of 425-degrees.

Put the cheese & creamed cheese into a microwave-safe dish. Microwave at 1-minute intervals until completely combined.

Stir the flour and egg into the dish until it is well-combined. Add any additional flour for consistency - until it stops sticking to your fingers.

With another medium-sized bowl, combine the chicken with sauce and set aside.

Cover a flat surface with plastic wrap or parchment paper and sprinkle with almond flour.

Spray a rolling pin to avoid sticking and use it to press the dough flat.

Make circle shapes out of this dough with a lid, a cup, or a cookie cutter. For excess dough, roll back up and repeat the process.

Portion out spoonful of filling into these dough circles but keep them only on one half.

Fold the other half over to close up into half-moon shapes. Press on the edges to seal them.

Lay on a lightly greased cooking sheet and bake for around 9 minutes until perfectly brown.

Nutrition: 96g Fat 74g Protein 1217 Calories

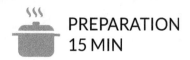

PREPARATION
15 MIN

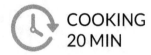

COOKING
20 MIN

SERVES
3

88. PEPPERONI AND CHEDDAR STROMBOLI

INGREDIENTS

- ▸ Mozzarella Cheese (1.25 cups)
- ▸ Almond Flour (0.25 cup)
- ▸ Coconut Flour (3 tablespoons)
- ▸ Italian Seasoning (1 teaspoon)
- ▸ Egg (1 large-sized; whisked)
- ▸ Deli Ham (6 ounces; sliced)
- ▸ Pepperoni (2 ounces; sliced)
- ▸ Cheddar Cheese (4 ounces; sliced)
- ▸ Butter (1 tablespoon, melted)
- ▸ Salad Greens (6 cups)

DIRECTIONS

First things first, bring the oven to a temperature of 400 degrees and prepare a baking tray with some parchment paper.

Use the microwave to melt the mozzarella until it can be stirred.

Mix flours & Italian seasoning in a separate small-sized bowl.

Dump in the melty cheese and stir together with pepper and salt to taste.

Stir in the egg and process the dough with your hands. Pour it onto that prepared baking tray.

Roll out the dough with your hands or a pin. Cut slits that mark out 4 equal rectangles.

Put the ham and cheese onto the dough, then brush with butter and close up, putting the seal end down.

Bake for around 17 minutes until well-browned. Slice up and serve.

Nutrition: 13g Fat 11g Protein 240 Calories

89. TUNA CASSEROLE

PREPARATION
15 MIN
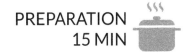

COOKING
10 MIN
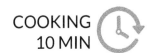

SERVES
4

INGREDIENTS

- Tuna in oil, sixteen ounces, drained
- Butter two tablespoons
- Salt, one-half teaspoon
- Black pepper, one teaspoon
- Chili powder, one teaspoon
- Celery, six stalks
- Green bell pepper, one
- Yellow onion, one
- Parmesan cheese, grated four ounces
- Mayonnaise, one cup

DIRECTIONS

Heat the oven to 400.

Chop the onion, bell pepper, and celery very fine and fry in the melted butter for five minutes.

Stir together with the chili powder, parmesan cheese, tuna, and mayonnaise.

Use lard to grease an eight by eight-inch or nine by a nine-inch baking pan.

Add the tuna mixture into the fried vegetables and spoon the mix into the baking pan.

Bake it for twenty minutes.

Nutrition: 953 Calories 83g fat 43g protein

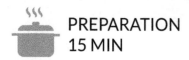

PREPARATION
15 MIN

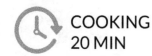

COOKING
20 MIN

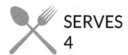

SERVES
4

90. BRUSSELS SPROUT AND HAMBURGER GRATIN

INGREDIENTS

- Ground beef, one pound
- Bacon, eight ounces, diced small
- Brussel sprouts, fifteen ounces, cut in half
- Salt, one teaspoon
- Black pepper; one teaspoon
- Thyme; one-half teaspoon
- Cheddar; cheese shredded one cup
- Italian seasoning; one tablespoon
- Sour cream; four tablespoons
- Butter; two tablespoons

DIRECTIONS

Heat the oven to 425.

Fry bacon and Brussel sprouts in butter for five minutes.

Stir in the sour cream and pour this mix into a greased eight by eight-inch baking pan.

Cook the ground beef and season with the salt and pepper, then add this mix to the baking pan.

Top with the herbs and the shredded cheese. Bake for twenty minutes.

Nutrition: 770 Calories 62g Fat 42g Protein

91. BOLOGNESE SAUCE

PREPARATION
15 MIN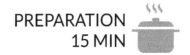

COOKING
45 MIN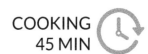

SERVES
10

INGREDIENTS

- ¼ c. dry white wine
- ¼ c. parsley, chopped
- ½ c. half & half
- 1 lg. white onion, diced
- 1 tbsp. butter, unsalted
- 2 lb. ground beef
- 2 med. carrots, diced
- 2 med. stalks, diced
- 3 bay leaves
- 4 oz. pancetta or bacon, chopped
- 56 oz. crushed tomatoes
- Sea salt & pepper, to taste

DIRECTIONS

Preheat huge pot over medium heat and brown the bacon or pancetta for about eight minutes.

Add the butter into the pot and stir in the celery and carrots. Cook until they're soft.

Add the ground meat to the pot, along with salt and pepper to taste. Break the meat up into chunks as it browns.

Add the wine to the sauce and allow it to reduce for a few minutes.

Add the crushed tomatoes to the pot and stir thoroughly, then add bay leaves, salt, pepper, and stir once more.

Cover and allow to simmer for twenty minutes.

Add the cream to the pot and pull the bay leaves out of the sauce.

Nutrition: 191 Calories 9g Fat 13g Carbohydrates

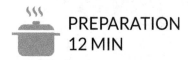

PREPARATION
12 MIN

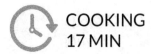

COOKING
17 MIN

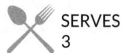

SERVES
3

92. SHEET PAN BURGERS

INGREDIENTS

- 24 oz. ground beef
- Sea salt & pepper, to taste
- ½ tsp. garlic powder
- 6 slices bacon, halved
- 1 med. onion, sliced into ¼ rounds
- 2 jalapeños, seeded & sliced
- 4 slices pepper jack cheese
- ¼ c. mayonnaise
- 1 tbsp. chili sauce
- ½ tsp. Worcestershire sauce

- 8 lg. leaves of Boston or butter lettuce
- 8 dill pickle chips

DIRECTIONS

Prep the oven to 425° Fahrenheit and line a baking sheet with non-stick foil.

Mix the salt, pepper, and garlic into the ground beef and form 4 patties out of it.

Line the burgers, bacon slices, jalapeño slices, and onion rounds onto the baking sheet and bake for about 18 minutes.

Garnish each patty with a piece of cheese and set the oven to boil.

Broil for 2 minutes, then remove the pan from the oven.

Serve one patty with 3 pieces of bacon, jalapeño slices, onion rounds, and desired amount of sauce with 2 pickle chips and 2 pieces of lettuce.

Nutrition: 608 Calories 46g Fat 5g Carbohydrates

93. ROASTED HERB GARLIC CHICKEN

PREPARATION
7 MIN
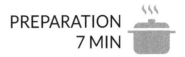

COOKING
14 MIN
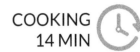

SERVES
5
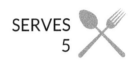

INGREDIENTS

- 1 ¼ lbs. chicken breasts, boneless & skinless
- 1 tbsp. garlic & herb seasoning mix
- 2 tsp. extra virgin olive oil
- Sea salt & pepper, to taste

DIRECTIONS

Heat a grill pan or your grill. Coat the chicken breasts in a little bit of olive oil and then sprinkle the seasoning mixture onto them, rubbing it in.

Cook the chicken for about eight minutes per side and make sure the chicken has reached an internal temperature of 165°. Serve hot with your favorite sides!

Nutrition: 187 Calories 6g Fat 1g Carbohydrates

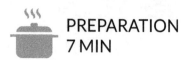

PREPARATION
7 MIN

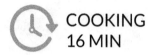

COOKING
16 MIN

SERVES
5

94. BLACKENED SALMON WITH AVOCADO SALSA

INGREDIENTS

- ▸ 1 tbsp. extra virgin olive oil
- ▸ 4 filets of salmon (about 6 oz. each)
- ▸ 4 tsp. Cajun seasoning
- ▸ 2 med. avocados, diced
- ▸ 1 c. cucumber, diced
- ▸ ¼ c. red onion, diced
- ▸ 1 tbsp. parsley, chopped
- ▸ 1 tbsp. lime juice
- ▸ Sea salt & pepper, to taste

DIRECTIONS

Preheat skillet over medium-high heat and warm the oil in it.

Rub the Cajun seasoning into the fillets, then lay them into the bottom of the skillet once it's hot enough.

Cook until a dark crust forms, then flip and repeat.

In a medium mixing bowl, combine all the ingredients for the salsa and set aside.

Plate the fillets and top with ¼ of the salsa yielded.

Nutrition: 445 Calories 31g Fat 10g Carbohydrates

PREPARATION
20 MIN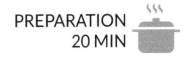

COOKING
15 MIN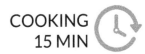

SERVES
4

95. CHICKEN PARMESAN

INGREDIENTS

- ¼ c. avocado oil
- ¼ c. almond flour
- ¼ c. parmesan cheese, grated
- ¾ c. marinara sauce, sugar-free
- ¾ c. mozzarella cheese, shredded
- 2 lg. eggs, beaten
- 2 tsp. Italian seasoning
- 3 oz. pork rinds, pulverized
- 4 lg. chicken breasts, boneless & skinless

DIRECTIONS

Preheat the oven to 450° Fahrenheit and grease a baking dish.

Place the beaten egg into one shallow dish. Place the almond flour in another. In a third dish, combine the pork rinds, parmesan, and Italian seasoning and mix well.

Pat the chicken breasts dry and pound them down to about ½" thick.

Coat the chicken in the almond flour, then coat in egg, then coat in crumb.

Heat a large sauté pan over medium-high heat and warm oil until shimmering.

Once the oil is hot, lay the breasts into the pan and do not move them until they've had a chance to cook. Cook for about two minutes, then flip as gently as possible then cook for two more. Remove the pan from the heat.

Place the breasts in the greased baking dish and top with marinara sauce and mozzarella cheese.

Bake for about 10 minutes.

Nutrition: 621 Calories 34g Fat 6g Carbohydrates

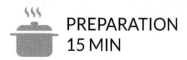

PREPARATION
15 MIN

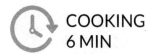

COOKING
6 MIN

96. TUNA BURGERS

SERVES
2

INGREDIENTS

- 1 (15-ounce) can water-packed tuna, drained
- ½ celery stalk, chopped
- 2 tablespoon fresh parsley, chopped
- 1 teaspoon fresh dill, chopped
- 2 tablespoons walnuts, chopped
- 2 tablespoons mayonnaise
- 1 organic egg, beaten
- 1 tablespoon butter
- 3 cups lettuce

. . . .

DIRECTIONS

For burgers: Add all ingredients (except the butter and lettuce) in a bowl and mix until well combined.

Make 2 equal-sized patties from mixture.

In a frying pan, warm up butter over medium heat and cook the patties for 2 minutes.

Carefully, flip the side and cook for about 2–3 minutes.

Divide the lettuce onto serving plates.

Top each plate with 1 burger and serve.

Nutrition: 631 Calories 39.9g Fat 0.3g Fiber 61g Protein

97. BEEF BURGERS

PREPARATION
15 MIN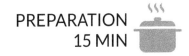

COOKING
6 MIN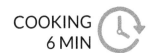

SERVES
2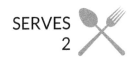

INGREDIENTS

- 8 ounces grass-fed ground beef
- Salt and ground black pepper, as required
- 1-ounce mozzarella cheese, cubed
- 1 tablespoon unsalted butter
- **Yogurt Sauce**
- 1/3 cup plain Greek yogurt
- 1 teaspoon fresh lemon juice
- ¼ teaspoon garlic, minced
- Salt, as required
- ½ teaspoon granulated erythritol

DIRECTIONS

In a bowl, add the beef, salt, and black pepper, and mix until well combined.

Make 2 equal-sized patties from the mixture.

Place mozzarella cube inside of each patty and cover with the beef.

In a frying pan, melt butter over medium heat and cook the patties for about 2–3 minutes per side.

Divide the greens onto serving plates and top each with 1 patty.

Serve immediately.

Meanwhile, for the yogurt sauce: place all the ingredients in a serving bowl and mix until well combined.

Divide patties onto each serving plate and serve alongside the yogurt sauce.

Nutrition: 322 Calories 19.8 Fat 29.8g Protein

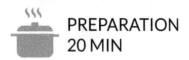 **PREPARATION**
20 MIN

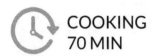 **COOKING**
70 MIN

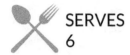 **SERVES**
6

98. LAMB MEATBALLS

INGREDIENTS

- 2 cups tomatoes, chopped
- 2 tablespoons fresh red chili
- 1 tablespoon fresh ginger
- ½ tablespoon fresh lime zest, grated
- ¼ cup organic apple cider vinegar
- 2 tablespoons red boat fish sauce
- 1 tablespoon fresh lime juice
- 2 tablespoons granulated erythritol
- ¼ teaspoon mustard powder
- ½ teaspoon dehydrated onion flakes
- ½ teaspoon ground coriander
- ½ teaspoon ground cinnamon
- ¼ teaspoon ground allspice
- 1/8 teaspoon ground cloves
- Salt, as required
- **Meatballs**
- 1-pound grass-fed ground lamb
- 1 tablespoon olive oil
- 1 teaspoon dehydrated onion flakes
- ½ teaspoon granulated garlic
- ½ teaspoon ground cumin
- ½ teaspoon red pepper flakes, crushed
- Salt, as required

DIRECTIONS

- **For chutney:**

Add all the ingredients in a pan over medium heat (except for cilantro) and bring to a boil.

Adjust the heat to low and simmer for about 45 minutes, stirring occasionally.

Remove from heat and set aside to cool.

Meanwhile, preheat your oven to 400°F.

Line a more massive baking sheet with parchment paper.

- **For meatballs:**

Incorporate all the ingredients and with your hands, mix until well combined.

Shape the mixture into desired and equal-sized balls.

Arrange meatballs into the prepared baking sheet in a single layer and bake for about 15–20 minutes or until done completely.

Serve the meatballs with chutney.

Nutrition: 184 Calories 8.1g Fat 1g Fiber

PREPARATION
15 MIN

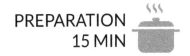

99. STUFFED ZUCCHINI

COOKING
18 MIN

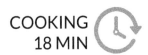

SERVES
8

INGREDIENTS

- ▸ 4 medium zucchinis
- ▸ 1 cup red bell pepper
- ▸ ½ cup Kalamata olives
- ▸ ½ cup fresh tomatoes
- ▸ 1 teaspoon garlic
- ▸ 1 tablespoon dried oregano
- ▸ ½ cup feta cheese, crumbled

DIRECTIONS

Preheat your oven to 350°F.

Grease a large baking sheet.

With a melon baller, spoon out the flesh of each zucchini half. Discard the flesh.

In a bowl, mix together the bell pepper, olives, tomatoes, garlic, oregano, salt, and black pepper.

Stuff each zucchini half with the veggie mixture evenly.

Arrange zucchini halves onto the prepared baking sheet and bake for about 15 minutes.

Now, set the oven to broiler on high.

Top each zucchini half with feta cheese and broil for about 3 minutes.

Serve hot.

Nutrition: 59 Calories 3.2g Fat 2.9g Protein

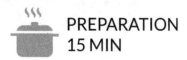

PREPARATION
15 MIN

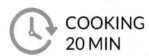

COOKING
20 MIN

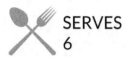

SERVES
6

100. STUFFED BELL PEPPERS

INGREDIENTS

- 2 teaspoons coconut oil
- 1-pound grass-fed ground beef
- 1 garlic clove, minced
- 1 cup white mushrooms
- 1 cup yellow onion
- ½ cup homemade tomato puree
- 3 large green bell peppers
- 1 cup water
- 4 ounces sharp cheddar cheese

DIRECTIONS

Warm up coconut oil in a wok over medium-high heat and sauté the garlic for about 30 seconds.

Add the beef and cook for about 5 minutes, crumbling with the spoon.

Add the mushrooms and onion and cook for about 5–6 minutes.

Stir in salt and black pepper and cook for about 30 seconds.

Pull away from the heat and mix in tomato puree.

Meanwhile, in a microwave-safe dish, arrange the bell peppers, cut-side down.

Pour the water in baking dish.

With a plastic wrap, cover the baking dish and microwave on high for about 4–5 minutes.

Remove from microwave and uncover the baking dish.

Dain the water completely.

Now in the baking dish, arrange the bell peppers, cut-side up.

Stuff the bell peppers evenly with beef mixture and top with cheese.

Microwave on High for about 2–3 minutes.

Serve warm.

Nutrition: 258 Calories 15.4g Fat 2.3g Fiber

101. SPINACH IN CREAMY SAUCE

PREPARATION
8 MIN
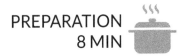

COOKING
17 MIN
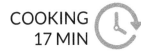

SERVES
5
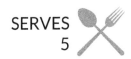

INGREDIENTS

- 2 tablespoons unsalted butter
- 1 small yellow onion, chopped
- 1 cup cream cheese, softened
- 2 (10-ounce) packages frozen spinach
- 3 tablespoons water
- 1 teaspoon fresh lemon juice

DIRECTIONS

Heat up butter in a wok over medium heat and sauté the onion for about 6–8 minutes.

Add the cream cheese and cook for about 2 minutes or until melted completely.

Stir in the spinach and water and cook for about 4–5 minutes.

Stir in the salt, black pepper, and lemon juice, and remove from heat.

Serve immediately.

Nutrition: 293 Calories 26g Fat 3.5g Fiber

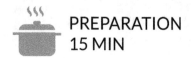

PREPARATION
15 MIN

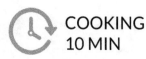

COOKING
10 MIN

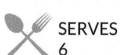

SERVES
6

102. CREAMY ZUCCHINI NOODLES

INGREDIENTS

- 1¼ cups heavy whipping cream
- ¼ cup mayonnaise
- 30 ounces zucchini, spiralized with blade C
- 3 ounces Parmesan cheese, grated
- 2 tablespoons fresh mint leaves
- 2 tablespoons butter, melted

DIRECTIONS

In a pan, add the heavy cream and bring to a boil.

Lower the heat to low and cook until reduced in half.

Add the mayonnaise, salt, and black pepper and cook until mixture is warm enough.

Add the zucchini noodles and gently, stir to combine.

Stir in the Parmesan cheese and immediately, remove from the heat.

Divide the zucchini noodles onto 4 serving plates and immediately, drizzle with the melted butter.

Nutrition: 249 Calories 23g Fat 1.7g Fiber

103. BROCCOLI WITH BELL PEPPERS

PREPARATION
15 MIN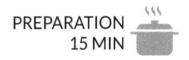

COOKING
10 MIN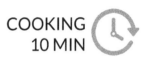

SERVES
6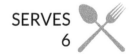

INGREDIENTS

- ▶ 2 tablespoons butter
- ▶ 2 garlic cloves, minced
- ▶ 1 large yellow onion, sliced
- ▶ 3 large red bell peppers
- ▶ 2 cups small broccoli florets
- ▶ 1 tablespoon low-sodium soy sauce
- ▶ ¼ cup homemade vegetable broth

DIRECTIONS

In a large wok, melt butter oil over medium heat and sauté the garlic for about 1 minute.

Add the vegetables and stir fry for about 5 minutes.

Stir in the broth and soy sauce and stir fry for about 4 minutes or until the desired doneness of the vegetables.

Stir in the black pepper and remove from the heat.

Serve hot.

Nutrition: 74 Calories 4.1g Fat 2.1g Protein

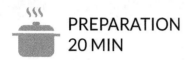

PREPARATION
20 MIN

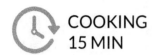

COOKING
15 MIN

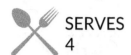

SERVES
4

104. SHRIMP IN CREAM SAUCE

INGREDIENTS

- **Shrimp**
- ½ ounce Parmigiano Reggiano cheese, grated
- 1 large organic egg
- 2 tablespoons almond flour
- ½ teaspoon organic baking powder
- ¼ teaspoon curry powder
- 1 tablespoon water
- 1-pound shrimp
- 3 tablespoons unsalted butter
- **Creamy Sauce**
- 2 tablespoons unsalted butter

- ½ of small yellow onion, chopped
- 1 garlic clove, finely chopped
- ½ cup heavy cream
- 1/3 cup cheddar cheese, grated
- 2 tablespoons fresh parsley, chopped

DIRECTIONS

- **For shrimp:**

Add all the ingredients (except shrimp) and butter in a bowl and mix until well combined.

Add the shrimp and coat with cheese mixture generously.

Melt the butter in a pan over medium heat and stir fry the shrimp for about 3–4 minutes or until golden-brown from all sides.

With a slotted spoon, transfer the shrimp onto a plate.

- **For sauce:**

Melt the butter in another pan over medium-low heat and sauté the onion for about 3–5 minutes.

Add garlic and sauté for about 1 minute.

Reduce the heat to low and stir in heavy cream and cheddar until well combined.

Cook for about 1–2 minutes, stirring continuously.

Stir in the cooked shrimps, parsley, salt, and black pepper, and cook for about 1–2 minutes.

Remove the pan of shrimp mixture from heat and transfer onto the serving plates.

Serve hot.

Nutrition: 410 Calories 29g Fat 32g Protein

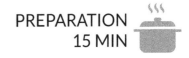

PREPARATION
15 MIN

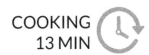

COOKING
13 MIN

SERVES
4

105. SCALLOPS IN GARLIC SAUCE

INGREDIENTS

- 1¼ pounds fresh sea scallops
- 4 tablespoons butter, divided
- 5 garlic cloves, chopped
- ¼ cup homemade chicken broth
- 1 cup heavy cream
- 1 tablespoon fresh lemon juice
- 2 tablespoons fresh parsley

DIRECTIONS

Sprinkle the scallops evenly with salt and black pepper.

Melt 2 tablespoons of butter in a large pan over medium-high heat and cook the scallops for about 2–3 minutes per side.

Flip the scallops and cook for about 2 more minutes.

With a slotted spoon, transfer the scallops onto a plate.

Now, melt the remaining butter in the same pan over medium heat and sauté the garlic for about 1 minute.

Pour the broth and bring to a gentle boil.

Cook for about 2 minutes.

Stir in the cream and cook for about 1–2 minutes or until slightly thickened.

Stir in the cooked scallops and lemon juice and remove from heat.

Garnish with fresh parsley and serve hot.

Nutrition: 435 Calories 33g Fat 25g Protein

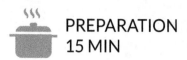

PREPARATION
15 MIN

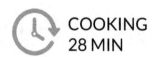

COOKING
28 MIN

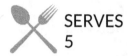

SERVES
5

106. BUTTER CHICKEN

INGREDIENTS

- 3 tablespoons unsalted butter
- 1 medium yellow onion, chopped
- 2 garlic cloves, minced
- 1 teaspoon fresh ginger, minced
- 1½ pounds grass-fed chicken breasts
- 2 tomatoes, chopped finely
- 1 tablespoon garam masala
- 1 teaspoon red chili powder
- 1 teaspoon ground cumin
- 1 cup heavy cream
- 2 tablespoons fresh cilantro

DIRECTIONS

Cook butter in a large wok over medium-high heat and sauté the onions for about 5–6 minutes.

Now, add in ginger and garlic and sauté for about 1 minute.

Add the tomatoes and cook for about 2–3 minutes, crushing with the back of spoon.

Stir in the chicken spices, salt, and black pepper, and cook for about 6–8 minutes or until desired doneness of the chicken.

Drizzle the heavy cream and cook for about 8–10 more minutes, stirring occasionally.

Garnish with fresh cilantro and serve hot.

Nutrition: 507 Calories 33g Fat 41g Protein

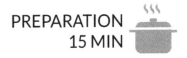

PREPARATION
15 MIN

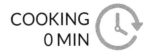

COOKING
0 MIN

SERVES
8

107. TOMATO & MOZZARELLA SALAD

INGREDIENTS

- 4 cups cherry tomatoes
- 1½ pounds mozzarella cheese
- ¼ cup fresh basil leaves
- ¼ cup olive oil
- 2 tablespoons fresh lemon juice
- 1 teaspoon fresh oregano
- 1 teaspoon fresh parsley
- 3 drops liquid stevia

DIRECTIONS

In a salad bowl, mix together tomatoes, mozzarella, and basil.

In a small bowl, add remaining ingredients and beat until well combined.

Place dressing over salad and toss to coat well.

Serve immediately.

Nutrition: 87 Calories 7.5g Fat 2.4g Protein

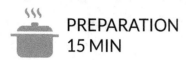

PREPARATION
15 MIN

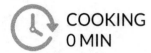

COOKING
0 MIN

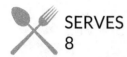

SERVES
8

108. CUCUMBER & TOMATO SALAD

INGREDIENTS

- **Salad**
- 3 large English cucumbers
- 2 cups tomatoes
- 6 cups lettuce
- **Dressing**
- 4 tablespoons olive oil
- 2 tablespoons balsamic vinegar
- 1 tablespoon fresh lemon juice

. . . .

DIRECTIONS

For salad: In a huge bowl, mix the cucumbers, onion, cucumbers.

For dressing: In a small bowl, add all the ingredients and beat until well combined.

Place the dressing over the salad and toss to coat well.

Serve immediately.

Nutrition: 86 Calories 7.3g Fat 1.1g Protein

PREPARATION
20 MIN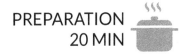

COOKING
16 MIN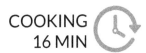

SERVES
8

109. CHICKEN & STRAWBERRY SALAD

INGREDIENTS

- 2 pounds grass-fed boneless skinless chicken breasts
- ½ cup olive oil
- ¼ cup fresh lemon juice
- 2 tablespoons granulated erythritol
- 1 garlic clove, minced
- 4 cups fresh strawberries
- 8 cups fresh spinach, torn

DIRECTIONS

Mix oil, lemon juice, erythritol, garlic, salt, and black pepper.

In a big resealable plastic bag, transfer the chicken and ¾ cup of marinade.

Seal bag and shake to coat well.

Refrigerate overnight.

Cover the bowl of remaining marinade and refrigerate before serving.

Preheat the grill to medium heat. Grease the grill grate.

Remove the chicken from bag and discard the marinade.

Place the chicken onto grill grate and grill, covered for about 5–8 minutes per side.

Remove chicken from grill and cut into bite sized pieces.

In a large bowl, add the chicken pieces, strawberries, and spinach, and mix.

Place the reserved marinade and toss to coat.

Serve immediately.

Nutrition: 356 Calories 21.4g Fat 34.2g Protein

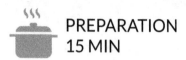

PREPARATION
15 MIN

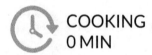

COOKING
0 MIN

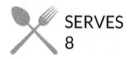

SERVES
8

110. SALMON SALAD

INGREDIENTS

- 12 hard-boiled organic eggs
- 1-pound smoked salmon
- 3 celery stalks
- 1 yellow onion
- 4 tablespoons fresh dill
- 2 cups mayonnaise
- 8 cups fresh lettuce leaves

DIRECTIONS

Incorporate all the ingredients (except the lettuce leaves) and gently stir to combine.

Cover and refrigerate to chill before serving.

Divide the lettuce onto serving plates and top with the salmon salad.

Serve immediately.

Nutrition: 539 Calories 49.2g Fat 19.4g Protein

CHAPTER 5. SOUP RECIPES

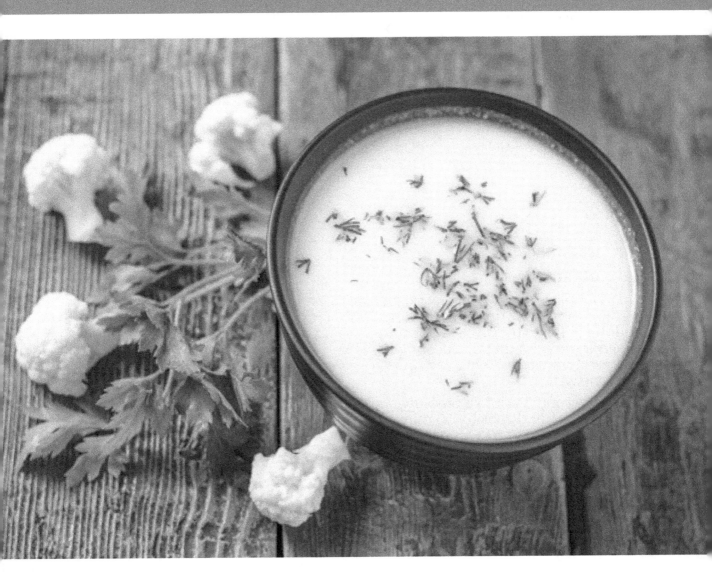

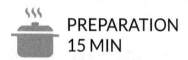

PREPARATION
15 MIN

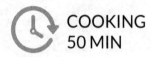

COOKING
50 MIN

SERVES
4

111. LAMB CURRY STEW

INGREDIENTS

- ▸ 1 tablespoon olive oil
- ▸ 1 small yellow onion, chopped
- ▸ 1½ pounds (680 g) boneless lamb shoulder, chopped
- ▸ 1 tablespoon curry powder
- ▸ 1½ cups chicken broth
- ▸ 2 cups chopped cauliflower

DIRECTIONS

Warm up olive oil in a nonstick skillet over medium-high heat until shimmering. Add the onion to the skillet and sauté for 4 minutes or until translucent. Add the remaining ingredients and sauté to combine well.

Transfer all of them into a pressure cooker. Put the lid on and cook for 50 minutes. Release the pressure, then remove the stew from the pressure cooker to a large bowl and serve warm.

Nutrition: 386 calories 14.7g total fat 2.1g fiber

PREPARATION
15 MIN

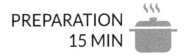

COOKING
0 MIN

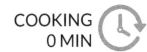

SERVES
6

112. COLD AVOCADO AND CRAB SOUP

INGREDIENTS

- ½ onion, diced
- ½ cup fresh cilantro, roughly chopped
- 1 cup watercress
- 1 cup heavy whipping cream
- 1 English cucumber, cut into chunks
- 2 avocados, diced
- 2 cups coconut water
- 2 teaspoons ground cumin
- Juice of 1 lime
- 1 pound (454 g) cooked crab meat

DIRECTIONS

Blend all the ingredients, except for the crab meat until smooth. Pour the soup in a large bowl. Add the crab meat into the soup and serve immediately

Nutrition: 298 calories 23.1g total fat 4.1g fiber

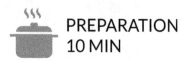

PREPARATION
10 MIN

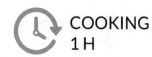

COOKING
1 H

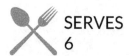

SERVES
6

113. SMOKED SALMON AND LEEK SOUP

INGREDIENTS

- 2 tablespoons extra-virgin olive oil
- ½ pound (227 g) smoked salmon
- 1 fish stock cube
- 1 leek, finely chopped
- 4 garlic cloves, crushed
- 1 small onion, finely chopped
- Salt, to taste
- 1 cup water
- 2 cups heavy whipping cream

DIRECTIONS

Brush the insert of the slow cooker with 2 tablespoons olive oil. Combine the salmon, stock cube, leek, garlic, onion, salt, and water in the slow cooker. Stir to mix well.

Put the slow cooker lid on and cook on LOW for 2 hours, then mix in the cream and cook for an additional 1 hour. Remove the soup from the slow cooker to a large bowl. Serve warm.

Nutrition: 219 calories 17.9g total fat 0.5g fiber

114. SPICY AND SOUR CHICKEN STEW

PREPARATION
10 MIN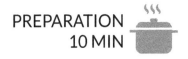

COOKING
80 MIN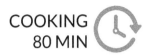

SERVES
6

INGREDIENTS

- ▸ 2 tablespoons extra-virgin olive oil
- ▸ 6 chicken thighs, skin on, boneless
- ▸ 1 chicken stock cube
- ▸ 1 red chili, finely chopped
- ▸ 1 small onion, finely chopped
- ▸ 2 limes
- ▸ 2 tins chopped tomatoes
- ▸ 3 garlic cloves, crushed
- ▸ 1 cup water

DIRECTIONS

Grease insert of the slow cooker with olive oil. Combine the remaining ingredients, except for the coriander, in the slow cooker. Stir to mix well.

Turn on slow cooker and cook on LOW for 6 hours. Put the stew to a big bowl. Top it with coriander and slice to serve.

Nutrition: 445 calories 32.2g total fat 1.1g fiber

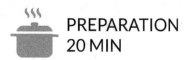

PREPARATION
20 MIN

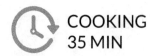

COOKING
35 MIN

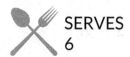

SERVES
6

115. CREAMY CHICKEN POT PIE SOUP

INGREDIENTS

- 2 tablespoons extra-virgin olive oil, divided
- 1 pound (454 g) skinless chicken breast
- 1 cup mushrooms, quartered
- 2 celery stalks, chopped
- 1 onion, chopped
- 1 tablespoon garlic, minced
- 5 cups low-sodium chicken broth
- 1 cup green beans, chopped
- ¼ cup cream cheese
- 1 cup heavy whipping cream
- 1 tablespoon fresh thyme, chopped

DIRECTIONS

Cook olive oil in a stockpot over medium-high heat until shimmering. Add the chicken chunks to the pot and sauté for 10 minutes or until well browned. Transfer the chicken to a plate. Set aside until ready to use.

Heat the remaining olive oil in the stockpot over medium-high heat. Add the mushrooms, celery, onion, and garlic to the pot and sauté for 6 minutes or until fork-tender.

Pour the chicken broth over, then add the cooked chicken chunks to the pot. Stir to mix well, and boil the soup. Adjust the heat to low. Simmer the for 15 minutes.

Mix in the green beans, cream cheese, cream, thyme, salt, and black pepper, then simmer for 3 more minutes. Remove the soup from the stockpot and serve hot.

Nutrition: 338 calories 26.1g total fat 2.2g fiber

PREPARATION
15 MIN

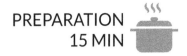

COOKING
75 MIN

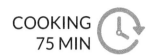

SERVES
6

116. SAUERKRAUT AND SAUSAGE SOUP

INGREDIENTS

- 1 tablespoon extra-virgin olive oil
- 1 pound (454 g) organic sausage, cooked and sliced
- 2 cups sauerkraut
- ½ teaspoon caraway seeds
- 1 sweet onion, chopped
- 1 tablespoon hot mustard
- 2 tablespoons butter
- 2 celery stalks, chopped
- 2 teaspoons minced garlic

- 6 cups beef broth
- ½ cup sour cream
- 2 tablespoons chopped fresh parsley, for garnish

DIRECTIONS

Brush insert of the slow cooker with olive oil. Combine the remaining ingredients, except for the sour cream and parsley, in the slow cooker. Stir to mix well.

Open the slow cooker and cook at low setting for 6 hours. Place the soup into a huge bowl, and mix in the sour cream. Top with parsley and serve warm.

Nutrition: 333 calories 28.1g total fat 2.1g fiber

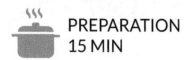

PREPARATION
15 MIN

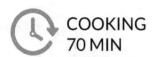

COOKING
70 MIN

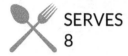

SERVES
8

117. JAMBALAYA BROTH

INGREDIENTS

- 1 tablespoon extra-virgin olive oil
- 6 cups chicken broth
- 1 (28-ounce / 794-g) can tomatoes, diced
- 1 pound (454 g) spicy organic sausage, sliced
- 1 cup cooked chicken, chopped
- 1 red bell pepper, chopped
- ½ sweet onion, chopped
- 1 jalapeño pepper, chopped
- 2 teaspoons garlic, minced
- 3 tablespoons Cajun seasoning
- ½ pound (227 g) medium shrimp, peeled,

deveined, and chopped
- ½ cup sour cream, for garnish
- 1 avocado, diced, for garnish
- 2 tablespoons chopped cilantro, for garnish

DIRECTIONS

Rub insert of the slow cooker with olive oil. Combine the chicken, sausage, broth, tomatoes, onion, jalapeño, bell pepper, Cajun seasoning, and garlic in the slow cooker. Stir to mix well.

Put the slow cooker lid on and cook on LOW for 6 hours. Add the shrimp and cook for an additional 30 minutes or until the fresh of the shrimp is opaque and a little white in color.

Transfer the soup into a large bowl. Add the avocado, sour cream, and cilantro, then stir to mix well before serving warm.

Nutrition: 402 calories 31.1g total fat 4.2g fiber

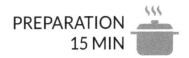

PREPARATION
15 MIN

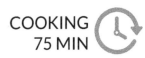

COOKING
75 MIN

SERVES
6

118. BEEF AND PUMPKIN STEW

INGREDIENTS

- 3 tablespoons extra-virgin olive oil, divided
- 1 (2-pound / 907-g) beef chuck roast
- ½ teaspoon salt
- ¼ teaspoon freshly ground black pepper
- ¼ cup apple cider vinegar
- ½ sweet onion, chopped
- 1 cup diced tomatoes
- 1 teaspoon dried thyme
- 1½ cups pumpkin, cut into 1-inch chunks
- 2 cups beef broth
- 2 teaspoons minced garlic
- 1 tablespoon chopped fresh parsley, for garnish

DIRECTIONS

Smear insert of the slow cooker with olive oil. Heat the remaining olive oil in a nonstick skillet. Add the beef to the skillet, and sprinkle salt and pepper to season.

Cook the beef for 7 minutes or until well browned. Flip the meat halfway through the cooking time. Put the cooked meat into the slow cooker, then add the remaining ingredients, except for the parsley, to the slow cooker. Stir to mix well.

Put the slow cooker lid on and cook on LOW for 8 hours or until the internal temperature of the beef reaches at least 145°F (63°C). Take out the stew from the slow cooker and top with parsley before serving.

Nutrition: 462 calories 34.1g total fat 3.2g fiber

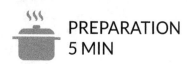 **PREPARATION**
5 MIN

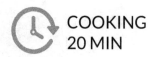 **COOKING**
20 MIN

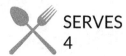 **SERVES**
4

119. CREAMY CAULIFLOWER AND CELERY SOUP WITH CRISP BACON

INGREDIENTS

- 2 tablespoons olive oil
- 1 onion, chopped
- 1 head cauliflower, cut into florets
- ¼ celery root, grated
- 3 cups water
- 1 cup white Cheddar cheese, shredded
- 1 cup almond milk
- 2 ounces (57 g) bacon, cut into strips

DIRECTIONS

Cook olive oil in a stockpot over medium heat until shimmering. Add the onion to the pot and sauté for 3 minutes or until translucent. Add the cauliflower florets and celery root to the pot and sauté for 3 minutes or until tender.

Pour the water into the pot, and sprinkle salt and black pepper to season. Stir well and boil. Low down the heat and put the lid on to cook for 10 minutes.

Use an immersion blender to mix the ingredients in the soup entirely, then mix in the cheese and almond milk. Fry the bacon in a nonstick skillet over high heat for 5 minutes or until curls and buckle. Turn the bacon halfway through the cooking time.

Divide the soup into four bowls and top with bacon. Serve hot.

Nutrition: 365 calories 27.2g total fat 22.7g protein

PREPARATION 5 MIN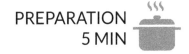

COOKING 25 MIN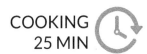

SERVES 4

120. SMOOTHIE GREEN SOUP

INGREDIENTS

- 2 tablespoons coconut oil
- ½ cup leeks
- 1 onion, chopped
- 1 garlic clove, minced
- 1 broccoli head, chopped
- 3 cups vegetable stock
- 1 bay leaf
- 1 cup spinach, blanched
- ½ cup coconut milk
- 2 tablespoons coconut yogurt, for garnish

DIRECTIONS

Heat up coconut oil in a stockpot over medium heat until shimmering. Add the leeks, onion, and garlic to the pot and cook for 5 minutes or until the onion is translucent. Add the broccoli to the pot and cook for 5 minutes more or until tender.

Pour the vegetable stock in the pot, and add the bay leaf. Close and boil the soup. Low down the heat and simmer for 10 minutes.

Add the spinach to the pot and simmer for 3 minutes. Use an immersion blender to mix the soup fully. Mix in the coconut milk, then season with salt and black pepper. Discard the bay leaf and divide the soup into four bowls, then top with coconut yogurt before serving.

Nutrition: 273 calories 24.6g total fat 4.6g protein

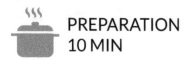

PREPARATION
10 MIN

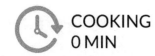

COOKING
0 MIN

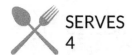

SERVES
4

121. RICH CUCUMBER AND AVOCADO SOUP WITH TOMATO

INGREDIENTS

- ½ cup plain Greek yogurt
- 1 garlic clove, minced
- 1 small onion, chopped
- 1 tablespoon cilantro, chopped
- 1½ cups water
- 2 limes, juiced
- 3 tablespoons olive oil
- 4 large cucumbers, chopped
- 2 chopped tomatoes, for garnish
- 1 chopped avocado, for garnish

DIRECTIONS

Put the all the ingredients, except for the avocado and tomatoes, in a food processor. Process for 2 minutes or until it has a mousse-like consistency.

Transfer the soup into a large bowl, then spread the avocado and tomatoes on top.

Wrap the bowl in plastic and refrigerate for 2 hours before serving or serve immediately.

Nutrition: 344 calories 26.2g fat 10.2g protein

122. BEEF STEW WITH MUSHROOMS AND ONIONS

PREPARATION 15 MIN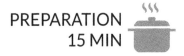

COOKING 30 MIN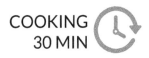

SERVES 6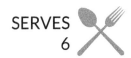

INGREDIENTS

- 2 lbs. beef sirloin
- 1 1/2 teaspoons sea salt
- 1/4 teaspoon ground black pepper
- 1/4 cup butter
- 2 lbs. chopped white mushrooms
- 1 medium yellow onion chopped
- 5 cloves garlic crushed
- 1/4 cup tomato paste
- 1 can 10 oz. cream of mushroom
- 4 cups beef broth

- 2 teaspoons dried parsley flakes
- 1/2 teaspoon dried oregano

DIRECTIONS

Season the beef. Let it stay for 10 minutes.

Cook 1 tablespoon butter in a Dutch oven or cooking pot. Cook beef for 3 to 5 minutes.

Remove the beef. Set Aside. Melt the remaining butter in the same cooking pot.

Once the butter melts, sauté the mushrooms, onions, and garlic. Cook until the mushrooms become soft.

Add the beef. Cook for 2 minutes.

Add the tomato paste, parsley, oregano, and beef broth. Stir and let boil. Cover and simmer 60 min.

Stir cream of mushroom for 2 to 3 minutes.

Turn the heat off. Transfer to a serving plate. Share and enjoy!

Nutrition: 452 Calories 2g Carbohydrates 49g Protein

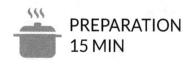

PREPARATION
15 MIN

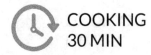

COOKING
30 MIN

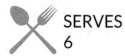

SERVES
6

123. TROUT BROILED WITH BUTTER AND SAUTÉED BOK CHOY

INGREDIENTS

- ▶ 1/2 tablespoon honey
- ▶ 1 tbsp. tamari
- ▶ 1 large garlic clove
- ▶ 3/4 tsp. chili powder
- ▶ 1 filet (6 oz.) trout fish
- ▶ 2 heads baby bok choy
- ▶ 1/2 tsp. sesame oil
- ▶ 1/4 tsp. hot pepper flakes

DIRECTIONS

Prep oven to 425 degrees Fahrenheit and line a baking sheet with parchment paper.

Scourge honey, half the tamari, minced garlic and chili powder.

Arrange rainbow trout skin side down onto parchment paper and season. Use a brush to spread the honey garlic mixture onto the fish.

Toss bok choy to a large mixing bowl and drizzle with the remaining tamari and sesame oil.

Situate bok choy to baking sheet and organize it around the rainbow trout.

Bake for 12 to 15 minutes.

Nutrition: 352 Calories 2g Carbohydrates 42.5g Protein

124. CAULIFLOWER SOUP WITH BACON OR TOFU

PREPARATION
20 MIN
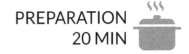

COOKING
60 MIN
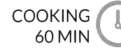

SERVES
8
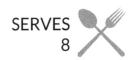

INGREDIENTS

- 1 medium head cauliflower
- 2 Tbsp extra virgin olive oil
- 2 carrots
- 3 celery stalks
- 2 shallots
- 3 garlic cloves
- 1 lb. silken tofu
- 3 Tbsp Kikkoman Traditionally Brewed Soy Sauce
- 8 cups vegetable broth

DIRECTIONS

Preheat broiler to 425.

Line a preparing sheet with tinfoil.

Spot cauliflower florets onto the preparing sheet and sprinkle with 1 Tbsp olive oil.

Broil cauliflower for around 40 minutes, flipping part of the way through cooking time, or until brilliant earthy colored and delicate. Expel from broiler.

In the interim, in an enormous soup pot, heat staying 1 Tbsp olive oil over medium warmth.

Include carrots, celery and shallots.

Sauté for around 5 minutes, mixing regularly, until vegetables perspire and relax however not earthy colored.

Include garlic and sauté one more moment.

Include tofu, separating it in the pot.

Include soy sauce and stock.

Bring to a stew.

When cauliflower is done simmered, add cauliflower to the pot.

Warm up to the point of boiling, at that point diminish to a stew for 5-10 minutes.

Expel pot from heat.

Carefully mix soup, utilizing a submersion blender, until smooth.

Spoon soup into bowls and top with chives and disintegrated bacon.

Present with a warm dried up entire baguette roll.

Nutrition: 541 Calories 4g Carbohydrates 34g Protein

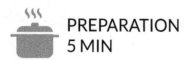

PREPARATION
5 MIN

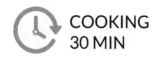

COOKING
30 MIN

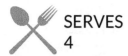

SERVES
4

125. GREEK EGG AND LEMON SOUP WITH CHICKEN

INGREDIENTS

- 4 cups of water
- ¾ lbs. cauli
- 1 lb. boneless chicken thighs
- 1/3 lb. butter
- Four eggs
- One lemon
- 2 tbsps. fresh parsley
- One bay leaf
- Two chicken bouillon cubes
- salt and pepper

DIRECTIONS

Slice your chicken thinly and then place it in a saucepan while adding cold water and the cubes and bay leaf. Let the meat simmer for 10 mins before removing it and the bay leaf.

Grate your cauli and place it in a saucepan. Add butter and boil for a few minutes.

Beat your eggs and lemon juice in a bowl, while seasoning it.

Reduce the heat a bit and add the eggs, stirring continuously. Let simmer but don't boil.

Return the chicken.

Nutrition: 582 Calories 49g Fats 31g Protein

126. CREAMY SEAFOOD SOUP

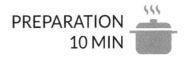

PREPARATION
10 MIN

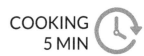

COOKING
5 MIN

SERVES
4

INGREDIENTS

▸ 1 tbsp avocado oil
▸ 2 garlic cloves, minced
▸ ¾ tbsp almond flour
▸ 1 cup (236 ml) vegetable broth
▸ 1 tsp dried dill
▸ 1 lb. (454 g) frozen mixed seafood
▸ Salt and black pepper to taste
▸ 1 tbsp plain vinegar
▸ 2 cups (454 g) cooking cream
▸ Fresh dill leaves to garnish

DIRECTIONS

Cook olive oil in a pot and sauté the garlic for 30 seconds or until fragrant.

Stir in the almond flour until brown.

Mix in the vegetable broth until smooth and stir in the dill, seafood mix, salt, and black pepper. Bring the soup to a boil and then simmer for 3 to 4 minutes or until the seafood cooks.

Add the vinegar, cooking cream and stir well.

Garnish with fresh dill and serve warm.

Nutrition: 401 Calories 36.6g Fat 0.1g Fiber

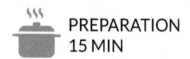

PREPARATION
15 MIN

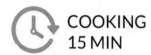

COOKING
15 MIN

SERVES
4

127. CREAMY CHICKEN AND MUSHROOM SOUP

INGREDIENTS

- 1 tbsp olive oil
- 2 chicken breasts
- Salt and black pepper to taste
- 2 cups cremini mushrooms
- 2/3 cup onions
- 1 tsp garlic powder
- 1 tsp dried parsley
- 1 tsp turmeric powder
- 1 tsp paprika
- 1 cup chicken broth
- 2 cups almond milk
- 1 cup heavy cream

- ½ cup cheddar cheese

DIRECTIONS

Cook olive oil in a pot over medium heat, season the chicken with salt, black pepper, and sear in the oil on both sides for 1 minute per side. Remove the chicken onto a plate and set aside.

Add the mushrooms, onions, and stir-fry for 5 minutes or until tender. Mix in the garlic powder, parsley, turmeric, and paprika. Cook for 1 minute.

Return the chicken to the pot, pour on the chicken broth and stir well. Boil then, simmer for 5 to 6 minutes or until the chicken cooks.

Use a fork to shred the chicken into strands. Whisk the almond milk, heavy cream, and simmer for 2 minutes and then, adjust the taste with salt and black pepper.

Dish the soup into serving bowls, top with the cheddar cheese and serve warm.

Nutrition: 1433 Calories 142g Fat 1g Fiber

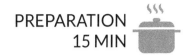

PREPARATION
15 MIN

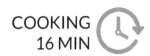

COOKING
16 MIN

SERVES
4

128. CREAMY ZUCCHINI SOUP

INGREDIENTS

- 1 tbsp coconut oil
- 1 medium yellow onion
- 3 garlic cloves
- 4 zucchinis
- 2 turnips
- ¼ cup fresh cilantro
- 2 tbsp chopped fresh mint
- 2 tsp curry powder
- ½ tsp cumin powder
- 2 cups vegetable broth
- Salt and black pepper to taste
- 1 ¼ cups almond milk
- 1 tbsp plain vinegar
- ¼ tsp red chili flakes

DIRECTIONS

Warm up coconut oil in a big pot and sauté the onion for 3 minutes or until softened. Stir in the garlic and cook for 30 seconds or until fragrant.

Mix in the zucchinis, turnips, cilantro, mint, curry powder, cumin powder, and vegetable broth. Season with salt, black pepper, and stir well. Boil then, simmer for 10 minutes.

With an immersion blender to puree the ingredients until smooth.

Stir in the almond milk, vinegar, and simmer for 2 minutes.

Topped with some mint leaves, red chili flakes and serve warm.

Nutrition: 653 Calories 71g Fat 1.3g Fiber

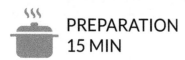

PREPARATION
15 MIN

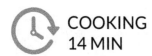

COOKING
14 MIN

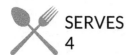

SERVES
4

129. CREAMY TAHINI ZOODLE SOUP

INGREDIENTS

- 2 tbsp coconut oil
- 2 tbsp butter
- ½ medium onion, chopped
- ½ cup sliced cremini mushrooms
- 1 garlic clove, minced
- 4 cups vegetable broth
- 4 tbsp coconut aminos
- 2 tbsp erythritol
- 2 tbsp tahini
- 4 tbsp heavy cream
- 4 zucchinis, spiralized

- **Topping:**
- 1 tbsp toasted sesame oil
- 1 tbsp chopped fresh scallions
- 1 tbsp toasted sesame seeds

DIRECTIONS

Warm up coconut oil and butter in a pot. Stir-fry the onion, and mushrooms for 5 minutes or until softened. Mix in the garlic and cook for 30 seconds or until fragrant.

Add the vegetable broth, coconut aminos, erythritol, tahini, heavy cream, and stir well. Boil the mix then, simmer for 5 minutes.

Mix in the zucchinis and cook for 3 minutes or until the zucchinis are tender.

Drizzle with the sesame oil, scallions, and sesame seeds.

Nutrition: 347 Calories 36g Fat 1.5g Fiber

130. ROASTED TOMATO AND CHEDDAR SOUP

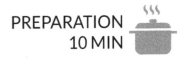

PREPARATION 10 MIN

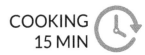

COOKING 15 MIN

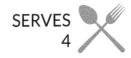

SERVES 4

INGREDIENTS

- 2 tbsp butter
- 2 medium yellow onions
- 4 garlic cloves, minced
- 5 thyme sprigs
- 8 basil leaves
- 8 tomatoes
- ½ tsp red chili flakes
- 2 cups vegetable broth
- Salt and black pepper to taste
- 1 cup grated cheddar cheese

DIRECTIONS

Melt the butter in a pot and sauté the onions and garlic for 3 minutes or until softened.

Stir in the thyme, basil, tomatoes, red chili flakes, and vegetable broth. Season with salt and black pepper.

Bring the soup to a boil and then, simmer for 10 minutes or until the tomatoes soften.

Puree the ingredients until smooth. Season well.

Dish the soup into serving bowls and garnish with the cheddar cheese and basil. Serve warm.

Nutrition: 346 Calories 31g Fat 15g Protein

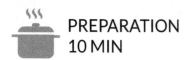

PREPARATION
10 MIN

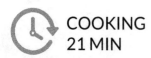

COOKING
21 MIN

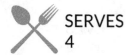

SERVES
4

131. GERMAN CHICKEN AND CHEESE SOUP

INGREDIENTS

- 1 tbsp olive oil
- ½ lb. ground chicken
- Salt and black pepper to taste
- 2 celery stalks
- 1 medium white onion
- 4 cups chicken stock
- 2/3 cup grated Gruyere cheese
- 9 1/3 oz crème fraiche
- 1 tsp nutmeg powder
- 1 tbsp fresh lemon zest

DIRECTIONS

Cook olive oil in a pot over medium heat and cook the chicken for 10 minutes or until no longer pink. Season with salt and black pepper.

Stir in the celery, onion and cook for 3 minutes or until softened.

Mix in the chicken stock, bring to a boil and then simmer for 8 minutes.

Add the cheese, crème fraiche, and nutmeg powder. Stir until the cheese melts. Season well.

Dash with lemon zest and serve warm.

Nutrition: 440 Calories 39g Fat 0.5g Fiber

PREPARATION
15 MIN
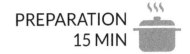

132. SWEET RUTABAGA CURRY SOUP

COOKING
19 MIN
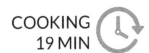

SERVES
4

INGREDIENTS

- 2 tbsp almond oil
- 2 tbsp butter
- 2 garlic cloves
- ¼ rutabaga
- 1 ½ cups coconut milk
- 1 ½ cups vegetable broth
- 1 tbsp red curry paste
- Salt and black pepper to taste
- Xylitol to taste
- 1 cup baby spinach

- 1 cup grated cheddar cheese
- 1 tbsp chopped fresh cilantro to garnish

DIRECTIONS

Heat the almond oil and butter in a pot and sauté the garlic until fragrant, 30 seconds.

Mix in the rutabaga, coconut milk, vegetable broth, red curry paste, salt, black pepper, and xylitol. Cover, bring to a boil, and then simmer for 10 to 15 minutes or until the rutabagas are tender.

Open and blend the soup until smooth.

Stir in the spinach, simmer for 2 to 3 minutes or until the spinach wilts. Season it well.

Dish the soup into serving bowls, top with the cheddar cheese, garnish with cilantro and enjoy warm.

Nutrition: 413 Calories 40g Fat 9.4g Protein

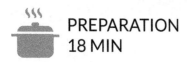

PREPARATION
18 MIN

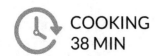

COOKING
38 MIN

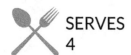

SERVES
4

133. TOMATO SOUP WITH GRILLED CHEESE SANDWICHES

INGREDIENTS

- 3 tbsp unsalted butter
- 1 tbsp almond oil
- 1 (7 oz) cans crushed tomatoes
- 2 medium white onions
- 1 ½ cups water
- Salt and black pepper to taste
- 1 tsp dried basil
- 8 low-carb bread slices
- 1 cup Gruyere cheese
- ½ cup grated Monterey Jack cheese
- 1 tbsp chopped fresh basil for garnish

DIRECTIONS

Cook 2 tablespoons of butter in a pot and mix in the tomatoes, onions, and water. Season with salt, black pepper, basil, and bring the mixture to a boil. Reduce the heat immediately and simmer for 30 minutes or until the liquid reduces by a third.

Meanwhile, melt a ¼ tablespoon of butter in a non-stick skillet over medium heat and lay in a bread slice.

Add a quarter each of both cheese on top and cover with another bread slice. Once the cheese starts melting and beneath the bread is golden brown, about 1 minute, flip the sandwich. Cook further for 1 more minute or until the other side of the bread is golden brown too.

Remove the sandwich to a plate and make three more in the same manner. Afterwards, diagonally slice each sandwich in half.

Dish the tomato soup into serving bowls when ready, garnish with the basil leaves, and serve warm with the sandwiches.

Nutrition: 285 Calories 25.2g Fat 12g Protein

PREPARATION
2 H

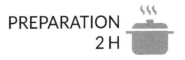

COOKING
11 MIN

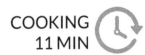

SERVES
4

134. COLD AVOCADO & GREEN BEANS SOUP

INGREDIENTS

- 1 tbsp butter
- 2 tbsp almond oil
- 1 garlic clove
- 1 cup green beans
- ¼ avocado
- 1 cup heavy cream
- ½ cup grated cheddar cheese
- ½ tsp coconut aminos
- Salt to taste

DIRECTIONS

Heat the butter and almond oil in a large skillet and sauté the garlic for 30 seconds. Add the green beans and stir-fry for 10 minutes or until tender.

Add the mixture to a food processor and top with the avocado, heavy cream, cheddar cheese, coconut aminos, and salt. Blend the ingredients until smooth.

Pour the soup into serving bowls, cover with plastic wraps and chill in the fridge for at least 2 hours.

Enjoy afterwards with a garnish of grated white sharp cheddar cheese

Nutrition: 301 Calories 30g Fat 4.8g Protein

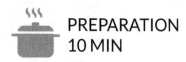

PREPARATION
10 MIN

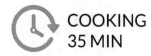

COOKING
35 MIN

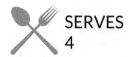

SERVES
4

135. THAI COCONUT SOUP

INGREDIENTS

- Three chicken breasts
- Nine oz. coconut milk
- Nine oz. chicken broth
- 2/3 tbsps. chili sauce
- 18 oz. water
- 2/3 tbsps. coconut aminos
- 2/3 oz. lime juice
- 2/3 tsp. ground ginger
- ¼ cup red boat fish sauce
- salt and pepper

DIRECTIONS

Slice up the chicken breasts thinly. Make them bite-sized.

In a large stockpot, mix your coconut milk, water, fish sauce, chili sauce, lime juice, ginger, coconut aminos, and broth. Bring to a boil.

Stir in chicken pieces. Then reduce the heat and cover pot, while simmering it for 30 mins.

Remove the basil leaves and season it.

Nutrition: 227 Calories 17g Fats 19g Protein

CHAPTER 6. APPETIZER AND SNACKS RECIPES

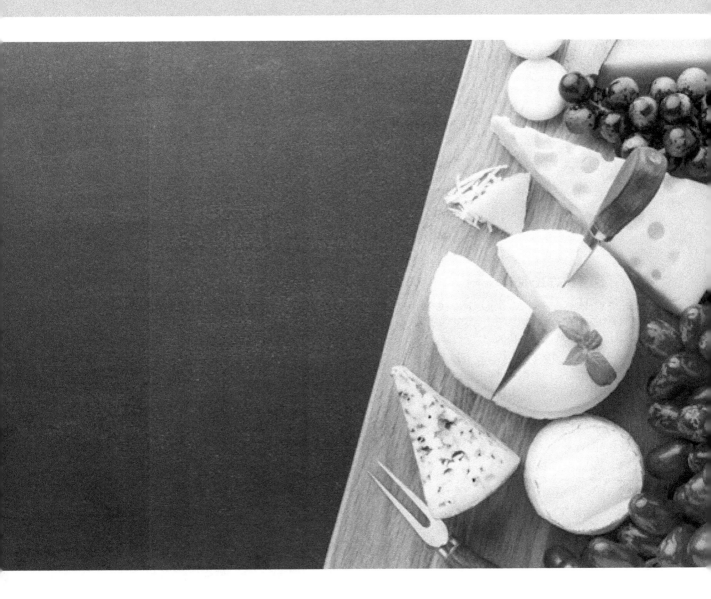

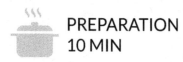

PREPARATION
10 MIN

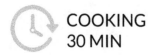

COOKING
30 MIN

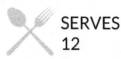

SERVES
12

136. PARMESAN CHEESE STRIPS

INGREDIENTS

- 1 cup shredded parmesan cheese
- 1 tsp dried basil

DIRECTIONS

Preheat the oven to 350 degrees Fahrenheit. Ready baking sheet by lining it with parchment paper.

Form small piles of the parmesan cheese on the baking sheet. Flatten it out evenly and then sprinkle dried basil on top of the cheese.

Bake for 5 to 7 minutes. Take it out, serve, and enjoy!

Nutrition: 31 calories 2g fat 2g protein

137. PEANUT BUTTER POWER GRANOLA

PREPARATION
10 MIN

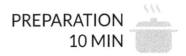

COOKING
40 MIN

SERVES
12

INGREDIENTS

- ▸ 1 cup almond flour
- ▸ 1 1/2 cups almonds
- ▸ 1 1/2 cups pecans
- ▸ 1/3 cup swerve sweetener
- ▸ 1/3 cup vanilla whey protein powder
- ▸ 1/3 cup peanut butter
- ▸ 1/4 cup sunflower seeds
- ▸ 1/4 cup butter
- ▸ 1/4 cup water

DIRECTIONS

Set oven to 300 degrees Fahrenheit and prep a baking sheet with parchment paper

Place the almonds and pecans in a food processor. Put them all in a large bowl and add the sunflower seeds, shredded coconut, vanilla, sweetener, and protein powder.

Melt the peanut butter and butter together in the microwave.

Mix the melted butter in the nut mixture and stir it thoroughly until the nuts are well-distributed.

Put in the water to create a lumpy mixture.

Scoop out small amounts of the mixture and place it on the baking sheet.

Bake for 30 minutes. Enjoy!

Nutrition: 338 calories 30g fat 9.6g protein

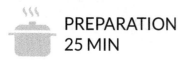

PREPARATION
25 MIN

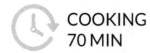

COOKING
70 MIN

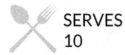

SERVES
10

138. HOMEMADE GRAHAM CRACKERS

INGREDIENTS

- 1 egg, large
- 2 cups almond flour
- 1/3 cup swerve brown
- 2 tsp cinnamon
- 1 tsp baking powder
- 2 tbsp melted butter
- 1 tsp vanilla extract

DIRECTIONS

Preheat the oven to 300 degrees Fahrenheit

Grab a bowl and whisk the almond flour, cinnamon, sweetener, baking powder, and salt. Stir all the ingredients together.

Put in the egg, molasses, melted butter, and vanilla extract. Stir until you get a dough-like consistency.

Roll out the dough evenly, making sure that you don't go beyond ¼ of an inch thick. Chop the dough into the shapes you want for cooking. Transfer it on the baking tray

Bake for 20 to 30 minutes until it firms up. Let it cool for 30 minutes outside of the oven and then put them back in for another 30 minutes. Make sure that for the second time putting the biscuit, the temperature is not higher than 200 degrees Fahrenheit.

Nutrition: 156 calories 13.35g fat 5.21g protein

PREPARATION
5 MIN

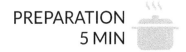

COOKING
10 MIN

SERVES
18

139. KETO NO BAKE COOKIES

INGREDIENTS

- 2/3 cup of all-natural peanut butter
- 1 cup of all-natural shredded coconut
- 2 tbsp real butter
- 4 drops of vanilla Lakanto

DIRECTIONS

Melt the butter in the microwave.

Take it out and put in the peanut butter. Stir thoroughly.

Add the sweetener and coconut. Mix.

Spoon it onto a pan lined with parchment paper

Freeze for 10 minutes

Cut into preferred slices. Store in an airtight container in the fridge and enjoy whenever.

Nutrition: 80 calories 5g fats 0.8g protein

PREPARATION
5 MIN

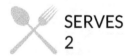

COOKING
20 MIN

SERVES
2

140. SWISS CHEESE CRUNCHY NACHOS

INGREDIENTS

- ½ cup shredded Swiss cheese
- ½ cup shredded cheddar cheese
- 1/8 cup cooked bacon pieces

DIRECTIONS

Set oven to 300 degrees Fahrenheit and prepare the baking sheet by lining it with parchment paper.

Start by spreading the Swiss cheese on the parchment. Sprinkle it with bacon and then top it off again with the cheese.

Bake until the cheese has melted. This should take around 10 minutes or less.

Allow the cheese to cool before cutting them into triangle strips.

Grab another baking sheet and place the triangle cheese strips on top. Broil them for 2 to 3 minutes so they'll get chunky.

Nutrition: 280 calories 21.8 fat 18.6g protein

141. HOMEMADE THIN MINTS

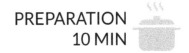

PREPARATION
10 MIN

COOKING
60 MIN

SERVES
20

INGREDIENTS

- 1 egg slightly beaten
- 1 3/4 cups almond flour
- 1/3 cup cocoa powder
- 1/3 cup swerve sweetener
- 2 tbsp butter melted
- 1 tsp baking powder
- 1/2 tsp vanilla extract
- 1/4 tsp salt
- **Coating:**
- 1 tbsp coconut oil

- 7 oz sugar free dark chocolate
- 1 tsp peppermint extract

DIRECTIONS

Preheat the oven to 300 degrees Fahrenheit. Ready baking sheet by lining it with parchment paper.

Grab a large bowl and combine the cacao powder, sweetener, almond flour, salt, and baking powder. Mix thoroughly before adding the already beaten egg, vanilla extract and butter.

Knead the dough and roll it on the parchment paper. Make sure it doesn't go beyond a thickness of ¼ inch.

Cut the cookie into your desired shapes. Combine and reroll, cut it up and again and repeat until nothing is left.

Bake for 25 minutes.

For the coating, melt the oil and chocolate in a bowl and stir until it's completely smooth. Use a microwave to do this or make sure of a pan placed in boiling water.

Once melted, stir in the peppermint extract.

Take the cookies and dip them in the coating, depending on your personal preferences. Allow it to dry on the surface and then refrigerate to keep it fresh.

Nutrition: 116 calories 10.41g fat 8g protein

PREPARATION
10 MIN

COOKING
30 MIN

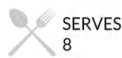

SERVES
8

142. MOZZARELLA CHEESE POCKETS

INGREDIENTS

- ▸ 1 large egg
- ▸ 8 pcs of mozzarella cheese sticks
- ▸ 1 ¾ cup mozzarella cheese
- ▸ ¾ cup almond flour
- ▸ 1 oz. cream cheese
- ▸ ½ cup of crushed pork rinds

DIRECTIONS

Start by grating the mozzarella cheese.

Scourge the almond flour, mozzarella, and the cream cheese. Microwave them for 3o seconds until you get that delicious gooey mixture.

Put in a large egg and mix the whole thing together. You should get a nice thick batch of dough.

Put the dough in between two wax papers and roll it around until you get a semi-rectangular shape

Cut them into smaller rectangle pieces and wrap them around the cheese sticks. Mold it depending on the shape you want.

Roll the stick onto crushed pork rinds.

Bake for 20 to 25 minutes at 400 degrees Fahrenheit.

Nutrition: 272 calories 22g fat 17g protein

143. NO BAKE COCONUT COOKIES

PREPARATION
5 MIN

COOKING
10 MIN

SERVES
8

INGREDIENTS

- 3 cups of unsweetened shredded coconut
- ½ cup sweetener
- 3/8 cup coconut oil
- 3/8 tsp. salt or to taste
- 2 tsp. vanilla
- Optional toppings: coconut shreds or finely-chopped nuts

DIRECTIONS

Position all the ingredients in a food processor without the optional toppings. You can also use the blender but try not to turn it too high because you'll end with a liquefied mix which won't produce the cookies in this recipe.

Remove and start forming them into the shape you want. Decorate as you want with the toppings.

Leave them to firm up for as long as necessary. This shouldn't take more than a few hours.

Nutrition: 329 calories 4.1g carbohydrates 2.1g protein

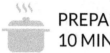

PREPARATION
10 MIN

COOKING
95 MIN

SERVES
4

144. CHEESY CAULIFLOWER BREADSTICKS

INGREDIENTS

- 4 eggs
- 4 cups of cauliflower riced
- 2 cups mozzarella cheese
- 4 cloves minced garlic
- 3 tsp. oregano

DIRECTIONS

Ready oven to 425 degrees Fahrenheit.

Line baking sheet by using parchment paper.

Situate cauliflower in a food processor or blender until finely chopped or when it resembles rice.

Put it in a covered bowl and microwave for just 10 minutes. Allow it to cool and if it's a little wet, make sure to drain it first before adding eggs, oregano, garlic, salt, pepper, and mozzarella. Mix them well.

Start separating the mixture into individual sticks – or really, just about any form you want.

Bake for 25 minutes. Pull out form the oven and sprinkle some more mozzarella on top while still hot. Put it back in the oven for just 5 minutes so that the cheese melts.

Nutrition: 99 calories 4g carbohydrates 13g protein

145. EASY PEANUT BUTTER CUPS

PREPARATION
10 MIN

COOKING
95 MIN

SERVES
12

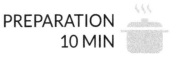

INGREDIENTS

- 1/2 cup peanut butter
- 1/4 cup butter
- 3 oz. cacao butter, chopped
- 1/3 cup powdered swerve sweetener
- 1/2 tsp vanilla extract
- 4 oz. sugar-free dark chocolate

DIRECTIONS

Prepare muffin tin with parchment paper.

Using low heat, melt the peanut butter, butter, and cacao butter in a saucepan. Stir them until thoroughly combined.

Add the vanilla and sweetener until there are no more lumps.

Carefully place the mixture in the muffin cups.

Refrigerate it until firm

Put chocolate in a bowl and set the bowl in boiling water. This is done to avoid direct contact with the heat. Stir the chocolate until completely melted.

Take the muffin out of the fridge and drizzle in the chocolate on top. Put it back again in the fridge to firm it up. This should take 15 minutes to finish.

Store and serve when needed.

Nutrition: 200 calories 19g fat 6g carbohydrates

PREPARATION
15 MIN

 COOKING
45 MIN

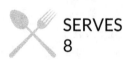 **SERVES**
8

146. SUGAR-FREE LEMON BARS

INGREDIENTS

- ½ cup butter, melted
- 1¾ cup almond flour, divided
- 1 cup powdered erythritol, divided
- 3 medium-size lemons
- 3 large eggs

DIRECTIONS

Prepare the parchment paper and baking tray. Combine butter, 1 cup of almond flour, ¼ cup of erythritol, and salt. Stir well. Place the mix on the baking sheet, press a little and put it into the oven (preheated to 350°F). Cook for about 20 minutes. Then set aside to let it cool.

Zest 1 lemon and juice all of the lemons in a bowl. Add the eggs, ¾ cup of erythritol, ¾ cup of almond flour, and salt. Stir together to create the filling. Pour it on top of the cake and cook for 25 minutes. Cut into small pieces and serve with lemon slices.

Nutrition: 4g Carbohydrates 26g Fat 272 Calories

PREPARATION
10 MIN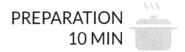

147. BANANA WAFFLES

COOKING
30 MIN

SERVES
4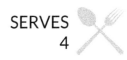

INGREDIENTS

- ▶ 4 eggs
- ▶ 1 ripe banana
- ▶ ¾ cup coconut milk
- ▶ ¾ cup almond flour
- ▶ 1 pinch of salt
- ▶ 1 tbsp. of ground psyllium husk powder
- ▶ ½ tsp. vanilla extract
- ▶ 1 tsp. baking powder
- ▶ 1 tsp. of ground cinnamon
- ▶ Butter or coconut oil for frying

DIRECTIONS

Mash the banana thoroughly until you get a mashed potato consistency.

Add all the other ingredients in and whisk thoroughly to distribute the dry and wet ingredients evenly. You should be able to get a pancake-like consistency

Fry the waffles in a pan or use a waffle maker.

You can serve it with hazelnut spread and fresh berries. Enjoy!

Nutrition: 4g carbohydrates 5g protein 155 calories

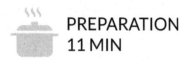

PREPARATION
11 MIN

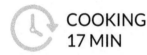

COOKING
17 MIN

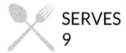

SERVES
9

148. KETO WAFFLES AND BLUEBERRIES

INGREDIENTS

- 8 eggs
- 5 oz. melted butter
- 1 tsp. vanilla extract
- 2 tsp. baking powder
- 1/3 cup coconut flour
- 3 oz. butter (topping)
- 1 oz. fresh blueberries (topping)

DIRECTIONS

Start by mixing the butter and eggs first until you get a smooth batter. Put in the remaining ingredients except those that we'll be using as topping.

Heat your waffle iron to medium temperature and start pouring in the batter for cooking

In a separate bowl, mix the butter and blueberries using a hand mixer. Use this to top off your freshly cooked waffles

Nutrition: 5g fiber 56g fat 575 calories

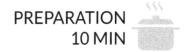

PREPARATION
10 MIN

COOKING
30 MIN

SERVES
4

149. BAKED AVOCADO EGGS

INGREDIENTS

- 2 avocados
- 4 eggs
- ½ cup bacon bits
- 2 tbsp. fresh chives, chopped
- 1 sprig of chopped fresh basil, chopped
- 1 cherry tomato, quartered
- Salt and pepper to taste
- Shredded cheddar cheese

DIRECTIONS

Select oven to 400 degrees Fahrenheit

Slice the avocado and remove the pits. Put them on a baking sheet and crack some eggs onto the center hole of the avocado. If it's too small, just scoop out more of the flesh to make room. Salt and pepper to taste.

Top with bacon bits and bake for 15 minutes.

Remove and sprinkle with herbs. Enjoy!

Nutrition: 271 calories 21g fat 5g fiber

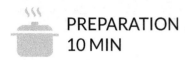

PREPARATION
10 MIN

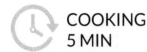

COOKING
5 MIN

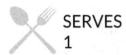

SERVES
1

150. MUSHROOM OMELET

INGREDIENTS

- 3 eggs, medium
- 1 oz. shredded cheese
- 1 oz. butter used for frying
- ¼ yellow onion, chopped
- 4 large sliced mushrooms
- Your favorite vegetables, optional

DIRECTIONS

Scourge eggs in a bowl. Add some salt and pepper to taste.

Cook butter in a pan using low heat. Put in the mushroom and onion, cooking the two until you get that amazing smell.

Pour the egg mix into the pan and allow it to cook on medium heat.

Allow the bottom part to cook before sprinkling the cheese on top of the still-raw portion of the egg.

Carefully pry the edges of the omelet and fold it in half. Allow it to cook for a few more seconds before removing the pan from the heat and sliding it directly onto your plate.

Nutrition: 5g carbohydrates 26g protein 520 calories

151. GARLIC PARMESAN CHICKEN WINGS

PREPARATION
10 MIN

COOKING
3 H

SERVES
2

INGREDIENTS

- ▶ Chicken Wings (2 lbs.)
- ▶ Garlic (4 cloves, chopped)
- ▶ Coconut Aminos (1/2 cup)
- ▶ Fish Sauce (1 tbsp.)
- ▶ Sesame Oil (2 tbsp.)

DIRECTIONS

Put wings into a large bowl, drain or pat to dry. In a small saucepan heat your ingredients, except wings. Remove from flame and add sesame oil.

Pour mixture over wings and stir. Cool and refrigerate overnight, you may stir occasionally as it marinates. Remove wings from marinade and bake wings at 375 degrees until they are done. Remove from heat and enjoy. Add your favorite side dish or have as is.

Nutrition: 738 Calories 39g Protein 66g Fats

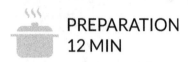

PREPARATION
12 MIN

COOKING
16 MIN

SERVES
6

152. CATFISH BITES

INGREDIENTS

- 1-pound catfish fillet
- 1 teaspoon minced garlic
- 1 large egg
- ½ onion, diced
- 1 tablespoon butter, melted
- 1 teaspoon turmeric
- 1 teaspoon ground thyme
- 1 teaspoon ground coriander
- ¼ teaspoon ground nutmeg
- 1 teaspoon flax seeds

DIRECTIONS

Cut the catfish fillet into 6 bites. Sprinkle the fish bites with the minced garlic. Stir it. Then add diced onion, turmeric, ground thyme, ground coriander, ground nutmeg, and flax seeds.

Mix the catfish bites gently. Prep air fryer to 360 F. Spray the catfish bites with the melted butter. Then freeze them. Put the catfish bites in the air fryer basket. Cook the catfish bites for 16 minutes. When the dish is cooked – chill it. Enjoy!

Nutrition: 140 Calories 13.1g Protein 8.7g Fats

153. SAVORY SALMON BITES

PREPARATION 2 H

COOKING 0 MIN

SERVES 12

INGREDIENTS

- Salmon trimmings (2 oz, smoked)
- Butter (2/3 cup, grass-fed, softened)
- Parsley (1 tbsp, chopped)
- Cheese (1 cup, mascarpone)
- Vinegar (1 tbsp, apple cider)

DIRECTIONS

Use a fork to smash the cheese and add the remaining ingredients. Form into small balls, and place on a tray lined with parchment paper. Refrigerate for approximately 2 hours. Serve.

Nutrition: 117 Calories 3g Protein 13g Fat

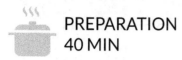

PREPARATION
40 MIN

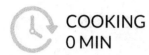

COOKING
0 MIN

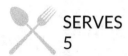

SERVES
5

154. HERBED CHEESE FAT BOMBS

INGREDIENTS

- Cream cheese (3.5 oz, full fat)
- Olives (4 pitted, green, chopped)
- Herbs (2 tsp, dried)
- Parmesan cheese (5 tbsp, grated)
- Salt and black pepper (to taste)
- Butter (1/4 cup, unsalted)
- Tomatoes (4 pieces, drained, chopped, sun dried)
- Garlic (2 cloves, crushed)

DIRECTIONS

Blend together the butter and the cream cheese. Transfer to a bowl. Add the next four ingredients. Season with salt and pepper, and mix.

Chill for 30 minutes. Form 5 balls out of the mixture. Cover each ball into the Parmesan cheese. Serve.

Nutrition: 164 Calories 3.7g Protein 17.1g Fat

PREPARATION
1 H
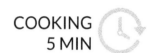

COOKING
5 MIN

SERVES
6

155. SAVORY FAT BOMBS

INGREDIENTS

- oz (100 g) cream cheese
- 1/4 cup (55 g/1.9 oz) butter, cubed
- 2 large (60 g/2.1 oz) slices of bacon
- 1 medium (15 g/0.5 oz) spring onion
- 1 clove garlic, crushed

DIRECTIONS

Add your cream cheese to a bowl with your butter. Leave uncovered to soften at room temperature. While that softens, set your bacon in a skillet on medium heat and cook until crisp. Allow it to cool then crumble into small pieces.

Add in your remaining ingredients to your cream cheese mixture and mix until fully combined. Spoon small molds of your mixture onto a lined baking tray (about 2 tbsp per mold). Then place to set in the freezer for about 30 minutes.

Set your Air Fryer to preheat to 350 degrees F. Put in the Air Fryer basket with gap in between and cook for 5 minutes. Cool to room temperature.

Nutrition: 108 Calories 2.1g Protein 11.7g Fats

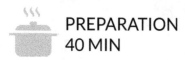

PREPARATION
40 MIN

COOKING
0 MIN

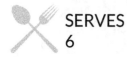

SERVES
6

156. PORK BELLY FAT BOMBS

INGREDIENTS

- Bacon (3 slices, cut in half widthwise)
- Mayonnaise (1/4 cup)
- Horseradish (1 tbsp, fresh, grated)
- Lettuce (6 leaves, for serving)
- Pork belly (5.3 oz, cooked)
- Dijon mustard (1 tbsp)
- Salt and pepper (to taste)

DIRECTIONS

Preheat the oven to 325°Fahrenheit. Cook the bacon slices on a baking sheet for a minimum of 30 minutes in the oven. Let cool.

Crush bacon into a dish and set aside. Shred the pork belly into a bowl and mix in the mustard, mayonnaise, and horseradish. Season with salt and pepper.

Divide the mixture into 6 mounds. Garnish with crumbled bacon

Nutrition: 263 Calories 3.5g Protein 126g Fat

PREPARATION
2 H

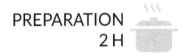

COOKING
0 MIN

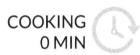

SERVES
6

157. CHEESY PESTO FAT BOMBS

INGREDIENTS

- ▶ Cream cheese (1 cup, full fat)
- ▶ Parmesan cheese (1/2 cup, grated)
- ▶ Pesto (2 tbsp, basil)
- ▶ Olives (10, green, sliced)

DIRECTIONS

Incorporate all the ingredients using a spatula. Serve as a dip with the cucumber (sliced) or other fresh vegetables.

You can also refrigerate for approximately 30 minutes, then create balls and roll into the Parmesan cheese. Serve.

Nutrition: 122 Calories 4.3g Protein 12.9g Fat

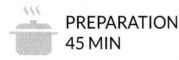

PREPARATION
45 MIN

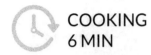

COOKING
6 MIN

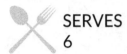

SERVES
6

158. VEGGIE AND CHEESE FAT BOMBS

INGREDIENTS

- Cream cheese (3.5 oz, full fat)
- Ghee (1 tbsp)
- Garlic (1 clove, peeled and finely chopped)
- Spinach (2 cups)
- Goat cheese (1/4 cup, hard, grated)
- Butter (1/4 cup, unsalted)
- Onion (1/2, chopped, peeled)
- Mushrooms (1/2 cup, dried porcini)
- Salt and pepper (to taste)

DIRECTIONS

Mix the butter and the cream cheese in a food processor. Sauté the onion and garlic with the ghee in a pan, over medium heat for approximately 3 minutes.

Add the dried mushrooms (chopped) and the spinach; cook for an additional 3 minutes. Set aside to cool. Mix the cream cheese and the butter with the spinach and cooled mushroom mixture. Season with salt and pepper. Cool for a minimum of 30 minutes. Create 5 balls out of the mix. Roll the balls onto the goat cheese. Serve.

Nutrition: 166 Calories 3.4g Protein 3.4g Fat

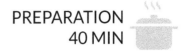

PREPARATION
40 MIN

COOKING
3 MIN

SERVES
4

159. CRISP BACON FAT BOMBS

INGREDIENTS

- Bacon slices (4 thick)
- Chile (1, green, seeded, chopped)
- Salt and pepper (to taste)
- Cream cheese (4 oz)
- Onion powder (1 tsp)

DIRECTIONS

Cook the bacon slices in a skillet for approximately 3 minutes. Let cool, then crumble. Reserve the bacon fat.

Combine the remaining ingredients in a bowl and add the bacon fat and mix. Shape mixture into 4 fat bombs. Refrigerate for 30 minutes. Roll the fat bombs in the bacon (crumbled). Serve.

Nutrition: 141 Calories 5.7g Protein 12.9g Fat

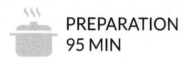

PREPARATION
95 MIN

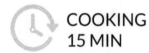

COOKING
15 MIN

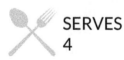

SERVES
4

160. BACON RANCH FAT BOMBS

INGREDIENTS

▸ Cream cheese (8 oz, full fat, softened)
▸ Bacon (2 slices)
▸ Ranch dressing (1 tbsp, dry mix)

DIRECTIONS

Preheat the oven to 375°Fahrenheit. Cook the bacon strips on a baking tray for approximately 15 minutes. Let cool, then crumble.

Add the cream cheese in a bowl, and sprinkle with the ranch dressing dry mix. Stir in the bacon and thoroughly mix. Form a ball out of 1 tablespoon of the mixture.

Repeat process to form 3 more bombs. Refrigerate for a minimum of 2 hours. Serve.

Nutrition: 419 Calories 11.4g Protein 39g Fat

PREPARATION
45 MIN

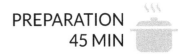

161. CHORIZO AND AVOCADO FAT BOMBS

COOKING
8 MIN

SERVES
4

INGREDIENTS

- ▸ Chorizo sausage (3.5 oz, diced, Spanish)
- ▸ Butter (1/4 cup, unsalted)
- ▸ Lemon juice (1 tbsp)
- ▸ Salt and cayenne pepper (to taste)
- ▸ Eggs (2 large, hard boiled, diced)
- ▸ Mayonnaise (2 tbsp)
- ▸ Chives (2 tbsp, chopped)
- ▸ Avocado (4, halves, pitted)

DIRECTIONS

Fry chorizo for 5 minutes in a hot pan. Set aside. Combine all the ingredients in a mixing bowl and season with salt and cayenne pepper to taste. Mash together with a fork. Refrigerate for approximately 30 minutes, and then fill each avocado half with ¼ of the mixture. Serve one-quarter of the mixture on top of each avocado half.

Nutrition: 419 Calories 11.4g Protein 38.9g Fat

PREPARATION
45 MIN

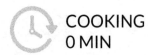

COOKING
0 MIN

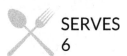

SERVES
6

162. TOMATO AND OLIVES FAT BOMBS

INGREDIENTS

- Butter (1/4 cup, unsalted)
- Tomatoes (1/4 cup, sun dried, chopped, drained
- Capers (2 tbsp, drained)
- Almonds (1/3 cup, flaked, raw or toasted)
- Cheese (1/4 cup, grated, Manchego)
- Olives (1/4 cup, green, pitted, sliced)
- Garlic (1 clove, crushed)
- Pepper (to taste)

DIRECTIONS

Beat cream cheese and butter in a food processor. Add the next five ingredients and season with pepper. Mix well.

Refrigerate for approximately 30 minutes. Make 6 balls out of the mixture. Roll each ball in the almond flakes. Serve.

Nutrition: 178 Calories 4.2g Protein 18g Fat

PREPARATION
45 MIN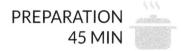

163. BRIE CHEESE FAT BOMBS

COOKING
3 MIN

SERVES
6

INGREDIENTS

- ▶ Cream cheese (2 oz, full-fat)
- ▶ Cheese (1/2 cup, Brie, chopped)
- ▶ Onion (1, white, diced)
- ▶ Paprika (1 tsp)
- ▶ Lettuce (6 leaves)
- ▶ Butter (1/4 cup, unsalted)
- ▶ Ghee (1 tbsp)
- ▶ Garlic (1 clove, minced)
- ▶ Salt and pepper (to taste)

DIRECTIONS

Mix the cream cheese and the butter in a food processor and transfer to a bowl. When finished mix in the Brie.

Add the onion and the garlic in a pan and cook for approximately 3 minutes over medium heat with the ghee. Let cool.

Once cooled, combine with the cheese and the butter mixture. Season with the spices and mix. Refrigerate for a minimum of 30 minutes. Make 6 fat bombs out of the mixture. Serve on lettuce leaves.

Nutrition: 158 Calories 3.3g Protein 16.2g Fat

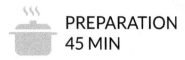

PREPARATION
45 MIN

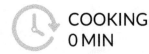

COOKING
0 MIN

SERVES
6

164. HAM & CHEESE FAT BOMBS

INGREDIENTS

- Cream cheese (3. Oz, full-fat)
- Cheese (1/4 cup, grated, cheddar)
- Ham (6 slices, Parma)
- Pepper (to taste)
- Butter (1/4 cup, unsalted)
- Basil (2 tbsp, fresh, chopped)
- Olives (6 large, green, pitted)

DIRECTIONS

Blend the cream cheese and the butter in a food processor. Add the Cheddar cheese and the basil, mix well. Season with pepper.

Refrigerate for a minimum of 30 minutes. Make 6 balls out of the mixture. Roll each ball with 1 slice of the Parma ham, top with 1 olive, piercing it with a toothpick. Serve.

Nutrition: 167 Calories 6.4g Protein 16.7g Fat

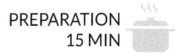

PREPARATION
15 MIN

COOKING
30 MIN

SERVES
4

165. CAULIFLOWER POPPERS

INGREDIENTS

- 4 cups cauliflower florets
- ¼ tsp. chili powder
- 2 tsp. olive oil
- Salt and ground black pepper, to taste

DIRECTIONS

Prepare the oven to 450 degrees F. Grease a roasting pan. In a bowl, add all ingredients and toss to coat well.

Transfer the cauliflower mixture into prepared roasting pan and spread in an even layer. Roast for about 25-30 minutes. Serve warm.

Nutrition: 46 Calories 2g Protein 2.5g Fats

CHAPTER 7. SIDES & SAUCES RECIPES

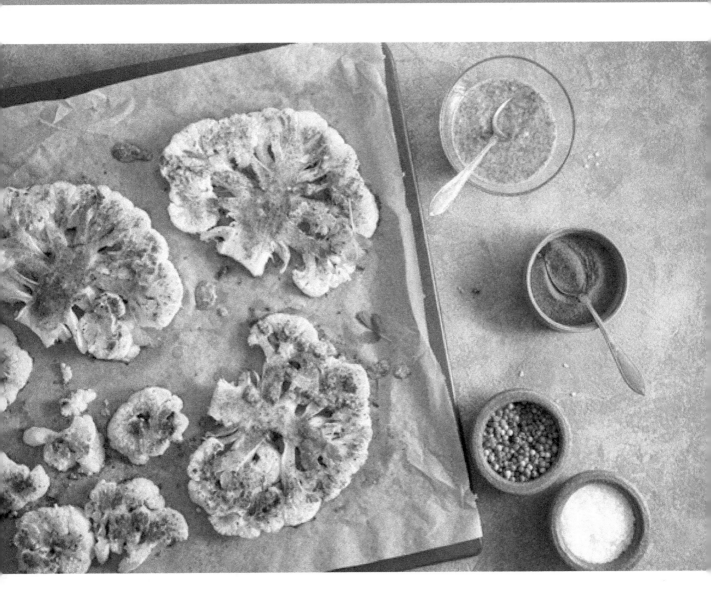

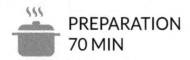

PREPARATION
70 MIN

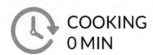

COOKING
0 MIN

SERVES
6

166. SIMPLE KIMCHI

INGREDIENTS

- ▸ 3 tablespoons salt
- ▸ 1-pound Napa cabbage, chopped
- ▸ 1 carrot, julienned
- ▸ ½ cup daikon radish
- ▸ 3 green onion stalks, chopped
- ▸ 1 tablespoon fish sauce
- ▸ 3 tablespoons chili flakes
- ▸ 3 garlic cloves
- ▸ 1 tablespoon sesame oil
- ▸ ½-inch fresh ginger

DIRECTIONS

Combine cabbage with the salt, massage well for 10 minutes, cover, and set aside for 1 hour.

In a bowl, mix the chili flakes with fish sauce, garlic, sesame oil, and ginger, and stir well.

Drain the cabbage well, rinse under cold water, and transfer to a bowl.

Add the carrots, green onions, radish, and chili paste and stir. Store for 2 days.

Nutrition: 160 Calories 3g Fat 2g Fiber

PREPARATION
6 MIN
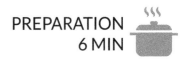

COOKING
19 MIN
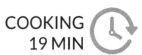

SERVES
5
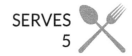

167. OVEN-FRIED GREEN BEANS

INGREDIENTS

- 2/3 Cup Parmesan cheese, grated
- 1 egg
- 12 ounces green beans
- Salt and ground black pepper, to taste
- ½ teaspoon garlic powder
- ¼ teaspoon paprika

DIRECTIONS

Incorporate the Parmesan cheese with salt, pepper, garlic powder, and paprika.

Scourge egg with salt and pepper. Dredge the green beans in egg, and then in the Parmesan mixture. Place the green beans on a lined baking sheet, place in an oven at 400°F for 10 minutes.

Nutrition: 114 Calories 5g Fat 7g Fiber

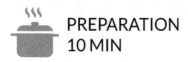

PREPARATION
10 MIN

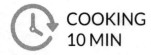

COOKING
10 MIN

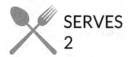

SERVES
2

168. CAULIFLOWER MASH

INGREDIENTS

- ¼ cup sour cream
- 1 small cauliflower head
- 2 tablespoons feta cheese, crumbled
- 2 tablespoons black olives

DIRECTIONS

Boil water with salt over medium heat, add the florets, cook for 10 minutes, take off the heat, and drain.

Return the cauliflower to the pot, add salt, black pepper, and sour cream, and blend using an immersion blender.

Add the black olives and feta cheese, stir and serve.

Nutrition: 100 Calories 4g Fat 2g Fiber

PREPARATION
10 MIN

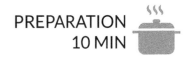

COOKING
10 MIN

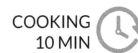

SERVES
4

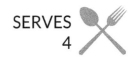

169. PORTOBELLO MUSHROOMS

INGREDIENTS

- 12 ounces Portobello mushrooms, sliced
- ½ teaspoon dried basil
- 2 tablespoons olive oil
- ½ teaspoon tarragon, dried
- ½ teaspoon dried rosemary
- ½ teaspoon dried thyme
- 2 tablespoons balsamic vinegar

DIRECTIONS

In a bowl, mix the oil with vinegar, salt, pepper, rosemary, tarragon, basil, and thyme, and whisk.

Add the mushroom slices, toss to coat well, place them on a preheated grill over medium-high heat, cook for 5 minutes on both sides, and serve.

Nutrition: 280 Calories 4g Fat 4g Fiber

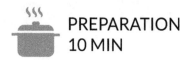

PREPARATION
10 MIN

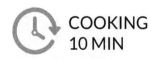

COOKING
10 MIN

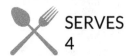

SERVES
4

170. BROILED BRUSSELS SPROUTS

INGREDIENTS

▸ 1-pound Brussels sprouts
▸ Salt and ground black pepper, to taste
▸ 1 teaspoon sesame seeds
▸ 1 tablespoon green onions, chopped
▸ 1½ tablespoons Sukrin gold syrup
▸ 1 tablespoon coconut aminos
▸ 2 tablespoons sesame oil
▸ 1 tablespoon sriracha

DIRECTIONS

Whisk sesame oil with coconut aminos, sriracha, syrup, salt, and black pepper.

Preheat pan over medium-high heat, add the Brussels sprouts, and cook them for 5 minutes on each side.

Add the sesame oil mixture, toss to coat, sprinkle sesame seeds, and green onions, stir again, and serve.

Nutrition: 110 Calories 4g Fat 4g Fiber

171. PESTO

PREPARATION
10 MIN
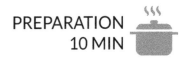

COOKING
0 MIN
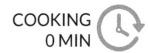

SERVES
4
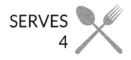

INGREDIENTS

- ½ cup olive oil
- 2 cups basil
- 1/3 cup pine nuts
- 1/3 cup Parmesan cheese, grated
- 2 garlic cloves, peeled and chopped

DIRECTIONS

Put the basil in a food processor, add the pine nuts, and garlic, and blend well.

Add the Parmesan cheese, salt, pepper, and the oil gradually and blend again until you obtain a paste. Serve with chicken or vegetables.

Nutrition: 100 Calories 7g Fat 3g Fiber

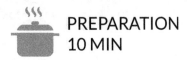

PREPARATION
10 MIN

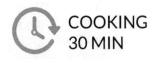

COOKING
30 MIN

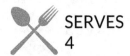

SERVES
4

172. BRUSSELS SPROUTS AND BACON

INGREDIENTS

- 8 bacon strips, chopped
- 1-pound Brussels sprouts
- A pinch of cumin
- A pinch of red pepper, crushed
- 2 tablespoons extra virgin olive oil

· ·

DIRECTIONS

Toss Brussels sprouts with salt, pepper, cumin, red pepper, and oil to coat.

Spread the Brussels sprouts on a lined baking sheet, place in an oven at 375°F, and bake for 30 minutes.

Heat a pan over medium heat, add the bacon pieces, and cook them until they become crispy.

Divide the baked Brussels sprouts on plates, top with bacon, and serve.

Nutrition: 256 Calories 20g Fat 6g Fiber

173. CREAMY SPINACH

PREPARATION
13 MIN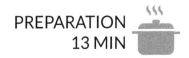

COOKING
17 MIN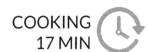

SERVES
3

INGREDIENTS

- 2 garlic cloves, peeled and minced
- 8 ounces of spinach leaves
- 4 tablespoons sour cream
- 1 tablespoon butter
- 2 tablespoons Parmesan cheese, grated

DIRECTIONS

Preheat pan with the oil over medium heat, add the spinach, stir and cook until it softens.

Add the salt, pepper, butter, Parmesan cheese, and butter, stir, and cook for 4 minutes.

Add the sour cream, stir, and cook for 5 minutes.

Divide between plates and serve.

Nutrition: 233 Calories 10g Fat 4g Fiber

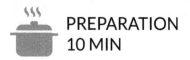

PREPARATION
10 MIN

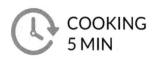

COOKING
5 MIN

SERVES
3

174. AVOCADO FRIES

INGREDIENTS

► 3 avocados
► 1½ cups sunflower oil
► 1½ cups almond meal

. . . .

DIRECTIONS

Scourge almond meal with salt, pepper, and cayenne. In different bowl, beat eggs with a pinch of salt and pepper.

Dredge the avocado pieces in egg and then in almond meal mixture. Heat a pan with the oil over medium-high heat, add the avocado fries, and cook them until they are golden.

Situate into paper towels, drain grease, and divide between plates and serve.

Nutrition: 200 Calories 43g Fat 4g Fiber

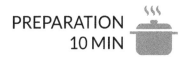

PREPARATION
10 MIN

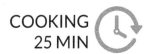

COOKING
25 MIN

175. ROASTED CAULIFLOWER

SERVES
6

INGREDIENTS

- ▸ 1 cauliflower head, separated into florets
- ▸ 1/3 cup Parmesan cheese, grated
- ▸ 1 tablespoon fresh parsley, chopped
- ▸ 3 tablespoons olive oil
- ▸ 2 tablespoons extra virgin olive oil

DIRECTIONS

In a bowl, mix the oil with garlic, salt, pepper, and cauliflower florets.

Toss to coat well, spread this on a lined baking sheet, place in an oven at 450°F, and bake for 25 minutes, stirring halfway. Add the Parmesan cheese, and parsley, stir and cook for 5 minutes.

Divide between plates and serve.

Nutrition: 118 Calories 2g Fat 3g Fiber

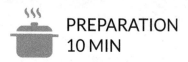

PREPARATION
10 MIN

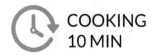

COOKING
10 MIN

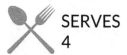

SERVES
4

176. MUSHROOMS AND SPINACH

INGREDIENTS

- 10 ounces spinach leaves
- 14 ounces mushrooms
- 2 garlic cloves
- ½ cup fresh parsley
- 1 onion
- 4 tablespoons olive oil
- 2 tablespoons balsamic vinegar

DIRECTIONS

Heat a pan with the oil over medium-high heat, add the garlic and onion, stir, and cook for 4 minutes.

Add the mushrooms, stir, and cook for 3 minutes.

Add the spinach, stir, and cook for 3 minutes.

Add the vinegar, salt, and pepper, stir, and cook for 1 minute.

Add the parsley, stir, divide between plates, and serve.

Nutrition: 200 Calories 4g Fat 6g Fiber

177. TZATZIKI

PREPARATION
10 MIN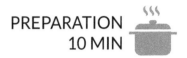

COOKING
0 MIN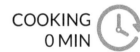

SERVES
8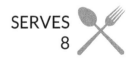

INGREDIENTS

- ½ c shredded cucumber, drained
- 1 tsp salt
- 1 T olive oil
- 1 T fresh mint, finely chopped
- 2 garlic cloves
- 1 c full-fat Greek yogurt
- 1 t lemon juice

DIRECTIONS

Place shredded cucumber on a strainer for an hour or squeeze out moisture through a cheesecloth.

Mix all ingredients in a medium bowl

Refrigerate.

Use as a vegetable dip, a dip for dehydrated vegetables, or a sauce for lamb, beef, or chicken. It is also a perfect accompaniment for fried summer squash.

Nutrition: 79 Calories 3g Carbohydrates 1g Protein

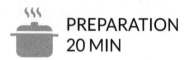

PREPARATION
20 MIN

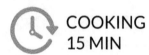

COOKING
15 MIN

SERVES
4

178. SATAY SAUCE

INGREDIENTS

- 1 can coconut cream
- 1 dry red pepper, seeds removed, chopped fine
- 1 clove garlic, minced
- ¼ c gluten-free soy sauce
- 1/3 c natural unsweetened peanut butter
- Salt and pepper

DIRECTIONS

Place all ingredients in a small saucepan.

Bring the mixture to a boil

Stir while heating to mix peanut butter with other ingredients as it melts.

After the mixture boils, turn down the heat to simmer on low heat for 5 to 10 minutes.

Remove from heat when the sauce is at the desired consistency.

Adjust seasoning to taste.

Nutrition: 312 Calories 7g Carbohydrates 7g Protein

PREPARATION
10 MIN

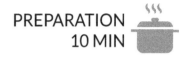

COOKING
5 MIN

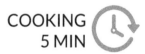

SERVES
8

179. THOUSAND ISLAND SALAD DRESSING

INGREDIENTS

- 2 T olive oil
- ¼ c frozen spinach, thawed
- 2 T dried parsley
- 1 T dried dill
- 1 t onion powder
- ½ t salt
- ¼ t black pepper
- 1 c full-fat mayonnaise
- ¼ c full-fat sour cream
- 2 t lemon juice

DIRECTIONS

Mix all ingredients in a small bowl.

Enjoy

Nutrition: 312 Calories 2g Carbohydrates 1g Protein

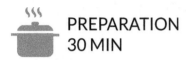

PREPARATION
30 MIN

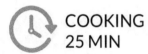

COOKING
25 MIN

SERVES
4

180. HOLLANDAISE SAUCE

INGREDIENTS

- 4 egg yolks
- 2 T lemon juice
- 1 ½ sticks of butter, melted
- Salt and pepper

· ·

DIRECTIONS

Heat water to boil in a saucepan.

Separate the eggs. Save the whites for another use.

Place the yolks in a heat-resistant bowl, either glass or stainless steel.

Carefully melt the butter in a saucepan without burning.

Place the bowl with the egg yolks over the simmering water to gently heat the eggs. Make sure the water is not touching the bottom of the bowl. The eggs need to be steamed, not cooked.

Add lemon juice to egg yolks.

Slowly stream the melted butter into the egg yolks while whisking. Start with a few drops of butter and then add a slow stream. Whisk the eggs the entire time until all the butter is added and the sauce has thickened.

Sprinkle with lemon juice, salt, and pepper.

Serve over poached eggs or cooked vegetables.

Nutrition: 566 Calories 1g Carbohydrates 3g Protein

PREPARATION
25 MIN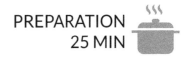

COOKING
20 MIN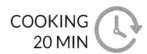

SERVES
2

181. LOW CARB STRAWBERRY JAM

INGREDIENTS

- Knox gelatin powder, three-fourths teaspoon
- Lemon juice, one tablespoon
- Water, one quarter cup
- Sugar replacement, one quarter cup
- Strawberries, diced, one cup

DIRECTIONS

Sprinkle the lemon juice with the gelatin and allow it to sit and thicken. Add the water, strawberries, and sugar replacement to a small pot and set it over medium heat.

As soon as this mixture begins to simmer then lower the heat and let it simmer for 20 minutes. Chop up the gelatin lemon juice mix and mix it in with the warm strawberries and let it dissolve.

Let the jam cool after removing the pan from the heat, then spoon the mix into a clean glass jar.

Nutrition: 57 Calories 1g Fat 0.6g Protein

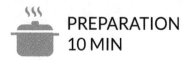

PREPARATION
10 MIN

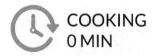

COOKING
0 MIN

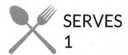

SERVES
1

182. PLAIN MAYONNAISE

INGREDIENTS

- ▸ Lemon juice, two teaspoons
- ▸ Olive oil, one cup
- ▸ Dijon mustard, one tablespoon at room temperature
- ▸ Egg yolk, one at room temperature

· ·

DIRECTIONS

Cream together the mustard and the egg yolk and then pour in the oil slowly while stirring to mix.

Add in the lemon juice and mix one last time and then let the mixture sit until it is thick.

Nutrition: 511 Calories 57g Fat 1g Protein

PREPARATION
1 H

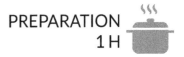

183. RANCH DIP

COOKING
0 MIN

SERVES
1

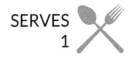

INGREDIENTS

- ▸ Ranch seasoning, two tablespoons
- ▸ Sour cream, one half cup
- ▸ Mayonnaise, one cup

DIRECTIONS

Mix all of the ingredients together and allow to chill for at least one hour before serving.

Nutrition: 241 Calories 26g Fat 1g Protein

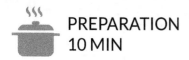

PREPARATION
10 MIN

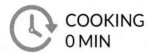

COOKING
0 MIN

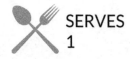

SERVES
1

184. AVOCADO SAUCE

INGREDIENTS

- Pistachio nuts, two ounces
- Salt, one teaspoon
- Lime juice, one quarter cup
- Garlic, minced, two tablespoons
- Water, one quarter cup
- Olive oil, two-thirds cup
- Avocado, one
- Parsley or cilantro, fresh, one cup

DIRECTIONS

Use a food processor or a blender to mix all of the ingredients together until they are smooth except the pistachio nuts and olive oil.

Add these at the end and mix well. If the mix is a bit thick add in a bit more oil or water.

Nutrition: 490 Calories 50g Fat 5g Protein

PREPARATION
1 H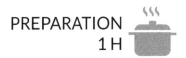

COOKING
0 MIN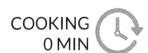

SERVES
1

185. BLUE CHEESE DRESSING

INGREDIENTS

- ▸ Parsley, fresh, two tablespoons
- ▸ Black pepper, one teaspoon
- ▸ Salt, one teaspoon
- ▸ Heavy whipping cream, one half cup
- ▸ Mayonnaise, one half cup
- ▸ Greek yogurt, three-fourths cup
- ▸ Blue cheese, five ounces

DIRECTIONS

Break the blue cheese up into small chunks in a large bowl. Stir in the heavy cream, mayonnaise, and yogurt.

Mix in the parsley, salt, and pepper and let the dressing sit for one hour, so the flavors mix well. This dressing will be good in the refrigerator for three days.

Nutrition: 477 Calories 47g Fat 10g Protein

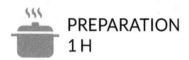

PREPARATION
1 H

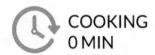

COOKING
0 MIN

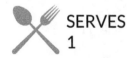

SERVES
1

186. SALSA DRESSING

INGREDIENTS

- Garlic, minced, one tablespoon
- Chili powder, one teaspoon
- Apple cider vinegar, three tablespoons
- Mayonnaise, two tablespoons
- Sour cream, two tablespoons
- Olive oil, one quarter cup
- Salsa, one half cup

DIRECTIONS

Mix all of the ingredients to a large bowl. Pour into a glass jar and let the dressing chill in the refrigerator for at least one hour.

Nutrition: 200 Calories 21g Fat 1g Protein

CHAPTER 8. DINNER RECIPES

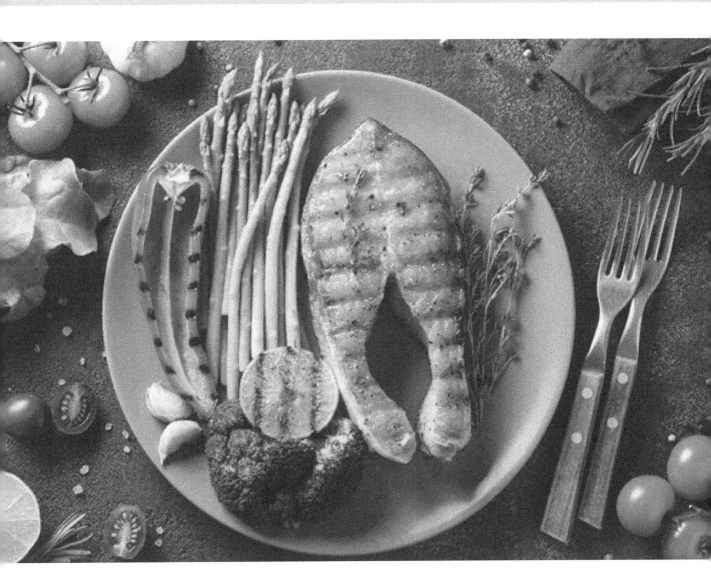

PREPARATION
13 MIN

COOKING
18 MIN

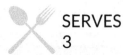

SERVES
3

187. PORK CHOPS WITH BACON & MUSHROOMS

INGREDIENTS

- 6 strips bacon, chopped
- 4 pork chops
- Salt and pepper to taste
- 2 cloves garlic, minced
- 8 oz. mushrooms, sliced
- 1 tablespoon olive oil
- 5 sprigs fresh thyme
- 2/3 cup chicken broth
- 1/2 cup heavy cream

DIRECTIONS

Cook bacon in a pan until crispy.

Transfer bacon on a plate.

Season the pork chops.

Cook the pork chops in bacon fat for 4 minutes per side.

Transfer pork chops on a plate.

Add the garlic and mushrooms in the pan.

Add the olive oil

Cook for 5 minutes.

Pour in the broth and let the mixture boil.

Stir in the heavy cream and reduce the heat to low.

Put the bacon and pork chops back to the pan.

Cook for 3 more minutes before serving.

Nutrition: 516 Calories 41g Fat 4.2g Carbohydrate

PREPARATION
10 MIN

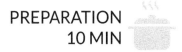

COOKING
20 MIN

SERVES
4

188. DELICIOUS PORK

INGREDIENTS

▸ A single pound of pork tenderloin
▸ A quarter cup of oil
▸ 3 medium shallots (chop them finely)

DIRECTIONS

Slice your pork into thick slices (go for about a half-inch thick).

Chop up your shallots before placing them on a plate.

Get a cast-iron skillet and warm up the oil

Press your pork into your shallots on both sides. Press firmly to make sure that they stick.

Place the slices of pork with shallots into the warm oil and then cook until it's done. The shallots may burn, but they will still be fine.

Make sure the pork is cooked through thoroughly.

Nutrition: 519 Calories 36g Fat 46g Protein

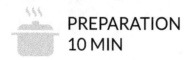

PREPARATION
10 MIN

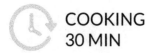

COOKING
30 MIN

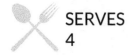

SERVES
4

189. GARLIC SHRIMP

INGREDIENTS

- 2 minced garlic cloves
- 2 whole garlic cloves
- Lemon juice
- 2 tablespoons olive oil
- 2 tablespoons of butter
- ¾ pounds shrimp
- A quarter of a teaspoon of paprika
- A quarter of a teaspoon of pepper flakes (red ones)
- 2 tablespoons of parsley that is chopped.

DIRECTIONS

Sprinkle your shrimp with a teaspoon of salt (fine grain sea salt) and let it sit for ten minutes.

Get a skillet.

Heat the butter with olive oil over a heat that is medium-high.

Add the flakes and garlic.

Sauté for half a minute.

Add your shrimp and cook until they have turned pink. This will take approximately two minutes. Stir constantly.

Add paprika and juice from the lemon.

Cook for another sixty seconds.

Nutrition: 260 Calories 18g Fat 24g Protein

190. PORK CHOP

PREPARATION
10 MIN

COOKING
30 MIN

SERVES
2

INGREDIENTS

▸ A dozen pork chop (boneless and thin cut)
▸ 2 cups of spinach (you should use baby spinach for this)
▸ 4 cloves of garlic
▸ A dozen slices provolone cheese

DIRECTIONS

Prep oven to a temperature of 350.

Pound the garlic cloves using a garlic press. The cloves should go through the press and into a small bowl.

Spread the garlic that you have made onto one side of the pork chops.

Flip half a dozen chops while making sure the garlic side is down.

You should do this on a baking sheet that is rimmed.

Divide your spinach between the half dozen chops.

Fold cheese slices in half.

Situate them on top of spinach.

Position the second pork chop on top of the first set, but this time make sure that the garlic side is up.

Bake for 20 minutes.

Cover each chop with another piece of cheese.

Bake another 15 minutes.

Your meat meter should be at 160 degrees when you check with a thermometer.

Nutrition: 436 Calories 25g Fat 47g Protein

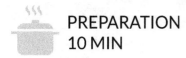

PREPARATION
10 MIN

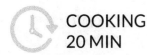

COOKING
20 MIN

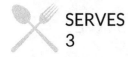

SERVES
3

191. CITRUS EGG SALAD

INGREDIENTS

- Half a dozen eggs (6)
- A single teaspoon of mustard (go with Dijon)
- 2 tablespoons of mayo
- A single teaspoon of lemon juice

DIRECTIONS

Place the eggs gently in a medium saucepan.

Add cold water until your eggs are covered by an inch.

Bring to a boil.

You should do this for ten minutes. Remove from your heat and cool. Peel your eggs under running water that is cold.

Put your eggs in a food processor. Pulse until they are chopped.

Stir in condiments and juice.

Nutrition: 22 Calories 19g Fat 13g Protein

192. CHOWDER

PREPARATION
10 MIN

COOKING
30 MIN

SERVES
4

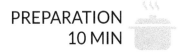

INGREDIENTS

- ▸ A single tablespoon of butter
- ▸ 5 minced garlic cloves
- ▸ An entire head of cauliflower (cut it into florets that are small)
- ▸ Half of a teaspoon of oregano (use dried)
- ▸ Half a cup of carrots that have been diced
- ▸ Half a cup of onions that have been diced
- ▸ A cup and a half of broth (use vegetable)
- ▸ A quarter cup of cream cheese

DIRECTIONS

Get a soup pot.

Heat your butter.

Add garlic and onions.

Sauté for a few moments.

Mix in the remaining ingredients to the pot.

Bring to a boil.

Slow the heat and put it on a simmer.

Cook for 15 minutes.

Shut off the flame.

Use a hand blender to blend the soup partly in the pot.

Switch the flame back on.

Add a cup of broth.

Add the cream cheese.

Simmer for 11 minutes then turn off the flame again.

Nutrition: 143 Calories 8.4g Fat 4.5g Protein

PREPARATION
10 MIN

COOKING
15 MIN

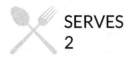

SERVES
2

193. CHICKEN QUESADILLAS

INGREDIENTS

- 1½ cups Mozzarella cheese, shredded
- 1½ cups Cheddar cheese, shredded
- 1 cup chicken, cooked and shredded
- 1 bell pepper, sliced
- ¼ cup tomato, diced
- 1/8 cup green onion
- 1 Tbsp extra-virgin olive oil

DIRECTIONS

Preheat the oven to 400°F. Use parchment paper to cover a pizza pan.

Combine your cheeses and bake the cheese shell for about 5 minutes.

Put the chicken on one half of the cheese shell. Add peppers, tomatoes, green onion and fold your shell in half over the fillings.

Return your folded cheese shell to the oven again for 4-5 minutes.

Nutrition: 6.1g Carbohydrates 40.5g Fat 52.7g Protein

194. SHRIMP LETTUCE WRAPS WITH BUFFALO SAUCE

PREPARATION 15 MIN

COOKING 20 MIN

SERVES 4

INGREDIENTS

- ▸ 1 egg, beaten
- ▸ 3 Tbsp butter
- ▸ 16 oz shrimp, peeled, deveined, with tails removed
- ▸ ¾ cup almond flour
- ▸ ¼ cup hot sauce (like Frank's)
- ▸ 1 tsp extra-virgin olive oil
- ▸ 1 head romaine lettuce, leaves parted, for serving
- ▸ ½ red onion, chopped
- ▸ celery, finely sliced
- ▸ ½ blue cheese, cut into pieces

DIRECTIONS

To make the Buffalo sauce, melt the butter in a saucepan, add the garlic and cook this mixture for 1 minute. Pour hot sauce into the saucepan and whisk to combine. Set aside.

In one bowl, crack one egg, add salt and pepper and mix. In another bowl, put the almond flour, add salt and pepper and also combine. Dip each shrimp into the egg mixture first and then into the almond one.

Take a large frying pan. Heat the oil and cook your shrimp for about 2 minutes per side.

Add Buffalo sauce.

Serve in lettuce leaves. Top your shrimp with red onion, blue cheese, and celery.

Nutrition: 8g Carbohydrates 54g Fat 33g Protein

PREPARATION
15 MIN

COOKING
8 MIN

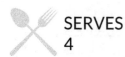

SERVES
4

195. WRAPPED BACON CHEESEBURGER

INGREDIENTS

- 7 oz bacon
- 1½ pounds ground beef
- ½ tsp salt
- ¼tsp pepper
- 4 oz cheese, shredded
- 1 romaine lettuce
- 1 tomato, sliced
- ¼ pickled cucumber, finely sliced

DIRECTIONS

Cook bacon and set aside. In different bowl, mix ground beef, salt, and pepper. Divide mixture into 4 sections, create balls and press each one slightly to form a patty.

Put your patties into a frying pan and cook for about 4 minutes on each side.

Top each cooked patty with a slice of cheese, several pieces of bacon, and pickled cucumber. Add a bit of tomato.

Wrap each burger in a big lettuce leaf.

Nutrition: 5g Carbohydrates 48g Protein 684 Calories

196. HEARTY LUNCH SALAD WITH BROCCOLI AND BACON

PREPARATION
10 MIN

COOKING
10 MIN

SERVES
5

INGREDIENTS

- 4 cups broccoli florets, chopped
- 7 slices bacon, fried and crumbled
- ¼ cup red onion, diced
- ¼ cup almonds, sliced
- ½ cup mayo
- ¼ cup sour cream
- 1 tsp white distilled vinegar
- 6 oz cheddar, cut into small cubes

DIRECTIONS

In a mixing bowl, combine the cheddar, broccoli, bacon, almonds, and onion. Stir these ingredients thoroughly.

In another bowl, combine the sour cream, mayo, vinegar, and salt. Stir the ingredients well and pour this mixture over your broccoli salad.

Nutrition: 20g Fat 12g Protein 267 Calories

PREPARATION
15 MIN

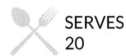

COOKING
15 MIN

SERVES
20

197. FATTY BURGER BOMBS

INGREDIENTS

- 1-pound ground beef
- ½ tsp garlic powder
- Kosher salt and black pepper
- 1 oz cold butter, cut into 20 pieces
- ½ block cheddar cheese, cut into 20 pieces

DIRECTIONS

Preheat the oven to 375°F. In a separate bowl, the mix ground beef, garlic powder, salt, and pepper. Use a mini muffin tin to form your bombs.

Put about 1 Tbsp of beef into each muffin tin cup. Make sure that you completely cover the bottom. Add a piece of butter on top and put 1 Tbsp of beef over the butter.

Place a piece of cheese on the top and put the remaining beef over the cheese. Bake your bombs for about 15 minutes.

Nutrition: 7g Fat 5g Protein 80 Calories

198. AVOCADO TACO

PREPARATION
10 MIN
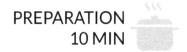

COOKING
15 MIN

SERVES
6

INGREDIENTS

- 1-pound ground beef
- 3 avocados, halved
- 1 Tbsp Chili powder
- ½ tsp salt
- ¾ tsp cumin
- ½ tsp oregano, dried
- ¼ tsp garlic powder
- ¼ tsp onion powder
- 8 Tbsp tomato sauce
- 1 cup cheddar cheese, shredded

- ¼ cup cherry tomatoes, sliced
- ¼ cup lettuce, shredded
- ½ cup sour cream

DIRECTIONS

Pit halved avocados. Set aside. Place the ground beef into a saucepan. Cook at medium heat until it is browned. Add the seasoning and tomato sauce. Stir well and cook for about 4 minutes.

Load each avocado half with the beef. Top with shredded cheese and lettuce, tomato slices, and sour cream.

Nutrition: 22g Fat 18g Protein 278 Calories

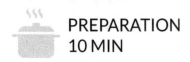

PREPARATION
10 MIN

COOKING
20 MIN

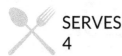

SERVES
4

199. TOFU SCRAMBLE WITH KALE & MUSHROOMS

INGREDIENTS

- 2 tablespoon ghee
- 1 cup sliced white mushrooms
- 2 cloves garlic, minced
- 16 oz. firm tofu, pressed and crumbled
- Salt and black pepper to taste
- ½ cup thinly sliced kale
- 6 fresh eggs

DIRECTIONS

Dissolve the ghee in a non-sticky skillet over medium heat and sauté the mushrooms for 5 minutes until they lose their liquid. Put garlic and cook for 1 minute.

Squeeze the tofu into the skillet, season with salt and black pepper. Cook with continuous stirring for 6 minutes. Introduce the kale in batches and cook to soften for about 7 minutes.

Crack the eggs into a bowl, whisk until well combined and creamy in color, and pour all over the kale. Use a spatula to immediately stir the eggs while cooking until scrambled and no runnier, about 5 minutes. Plate, and serve with low carb crusted bread.

Nutrition: 469 calories 39g Fat 25g Protein

PREPARATION
5 MIN

COOKING
30 MIN

SERVES
4

200. EGG IN A CHEESY SPINACH NESTS

INGREDIENTS

- 2 tablespoon olive oil
- 1 clove garlic, grated
- ½ lb. spinach, chopped
- Salt and black pepper to taste
- 2 tablespoon shredded Parmesan cheese
- 2 tablespoon shredded Gouda cheese
- 4 eggs

DIRECTIONS

Preheat oven to 350°F. Warm the oil in a non-stick skillet over medium heat; add the garlic and sauté until softened for 2 minutes. Add the spinach to wilt for about 5 minutes, and season with salt and black pepper. Allow cooling.

Grease a baking sheet with cooking spray; mold 4 (firm and separate) spinach nests on the sheet, and crack an egg into each nest. Sprinkle with Parmesan and Gouda cheese.

Bake for 15 minutes just until the egg whites have set and the yolks are still runny. Plate the nests and serve right away with low carb toasts and coffee.

Nutrition: 230 Calories 18g Fat 12g Protein

PREPARATION
10 MIN

COOKING
30 MIN

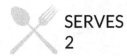

SERVES
2

201. BACON & CHEESE PESTO MUG CAKES

INGREDIENTS

- ¼ cup flax meal
- 1 egg
- 2 tablespoon heavy cream
- 2 tablespoon pesto
- ¼ cup almond flour
- ¼ teaspoon baking soda
- **Filling:**
- 2 tbsp. cream cheese
- 4 slices bacon
- ½ medium avocado, sliced

DIRECTIONS

Mix together the dry muffin ingredients in a bowl. Add egg, heavy cream, and pesto, and whisk well with a fork. Season with salt and pepper. Divide the mixture between two ramekins.

Place in the microwave and cook for 60-90 seconds. Leave to cool slightly before filling.

Meanwhile, in a skillet, over medium heat, cook the bacon slices until crispy. Transfer to paper towels to soak up excess fat; set aside. Invert the muffins onto a plate and cut in half, crosswise. To assemble the sandwiches: spread cream cheese and top with bacon and avocado slices.

Nutrition: 511 Calories 38.2g Fat 16.4g Protein

202. CHICKEN PAN WITH VEGGIES AND PESTO

PREPARATION
10 MIN

COOKING
20 MIN

SERVES
4

INGREDIENTS

- 2 Tbsp olive oil
- 1-pound chicken thighs
- ¾ cup oil-packed sun-dried tomatoes
- 1-pound asparagus ends
- ¼ cup basil pesto
- 1 cup cherry tomatoes, red and yellow

DIRECTIONS

Cook olive oil in a frying pan over medium-high heat.

Put salt on the chicken slices and the put into a skillet, add the sun-dried tomatoes and fry for 5-10 minutes. Remove the chicken slices and season with salt. Add asparagus to the skillet. Cook for additional 5-10 minutes.

Position the chicken back in the skillet, pour in the pesto and whisk. Fry for 1-2 minutes. Remove from the heat. Add the halved cherry tomatoes and pesto. Stir well and serve.

Nutrition: 32g Fat 2g Protein 423 Calories

PREPARATION
15 MIN

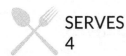

COOKING
20 MIN

SERVES
4

203. CABBAGE SOUP WITH BEEF

INGREDIENTS

- 2 Tbsp olive oil
- 1 medium onion, chopped
- 1-pound fillet steak, cut into pieces
- ½ stalk celery, chopped
- 1 carrot, peeled and diced
- ½ head small green cabbage
- 2 cloves garlic, minced
- 4 cups beef broth
- 2 Tbsp fresh parsley, chopped
- 1 tsp dried thyme
- 1 tsp dried rosemary
- 1 tsp garlic powder

DIRECTIONS

Heat oil in a pot (use medium heat). Add the beef and cook until it is browned. Put the onion into the pot and boil for 3-4 minutes.

Add the celery and carrot. Stir well and cook for about 3-4 minutes. Add the cabbage and boil until it starts softening. Add garlic and simmer for about 1 minute.

Pour the broth into the pot. Add the parsley and garlic powder. Mix thoroughly and reduce heat to medium-low.

Cook for 10-15 minutes.

Nutrition: 11g Fat 12g Protein 177 Calories

204. CAULIFLOWER RICE SOUP WITH CHICKEN

PREPARATION
10 MIN

COOKING
1 H

SERVES
5

INGREDIENTS

- 2 ½ pounds chicken breasts
- 8 Tbsp butter
- ¼ cup celery, chopped
- ½ cup onion, chopped
- 4 cloves garlic, minced
- 2 12-ounce packages steamed cauliflower rice
- 1 Tbsp parsley, chopped
- 2 tsp poultry seasoning
- ½ cup carrot, grated
- ¾ tsp rosemary
- 1 tsp salt
- ¾ tsp pepper
- 4 ounces cream cheese
- 4 ¾ cup chicken broth

DIRECTIONS

Put shredded chicken breasts into a saucepan and pour in the chicken broth. Add salt and pepper. Cook for 1 hour.

In another pot, melt the butter. Add the onion, garlic, and celery. Sauté until the mix is translucent. Add the rice cauliflower, rosemary, and carrot. Mix and cook for 7 minutes.

Mix chicken breasts and broth to the cauliflower mix. Put the lid on and simmer for 15 minutes.

Nutrition: 30g Fat 27g Protein 415 Calories

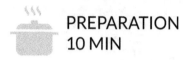

PREPARATION
10 MIN

COOKING
20 MIN

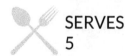

SERVES
5

205. QUICK PUMPKIN SOUP

INGREDIENTS

- 1 cup coconut milk
- 2 cups chicken broth
- 6 cups baked pumpkin
- 1 tsp garlic powder
- 1 tsp ground cinnamon
- 1 tsp dried ginger
- 1 tsp nutmeg
- 1 tsp paprika
- Sour cream or coconut yogurt, for topping
- Pumpkin seeds, toasted, for topping

DIRECTIONS

Combine the coconut milk, broth, baked pumpkin, and spices in a soup pan (use medium heat). Stir occasionally and simmer for 15 minutes.

With an immersion blender, blend the soup mix for 1 minute.

Top with sour cream or coconut yogurt and pumpkin seeds.

Nutrition: 9.8g Fat 3.1g Protein 123 Calories

206. FRESH AVOCADO SOUP

PREPARATION 5 MIN

COOKING 10 MIN

SERVES 2

INGREDIENTS

- 1 ripe avocado
- 2 romaine lettuce leaves
- 1 cup coconut milk, chilled
- 1 Tbsp lime juice
- 20 fresh mint leaves

DIRECTIONS

Mix all your ingredients thoroughly in a blender.

Chill in the fridge for 5-10 minutes.

Nutrition: 26g Fat 4g Protein 280 Calories

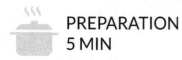

PREPARATION
5 MIN

COOKING
15 MIN

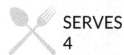

SERVES
4

207. CREAMY GARLIC CHICKEN

INGREDIENTS

- 4 chicken breasts
- 1 tsp garlic powder
- 1 tsp paprika
- 2 Tbsp butter
- 1 tsp salt
- 1 cup heavy cream
- ½ cup sun-dried tomatoes
- 2 cloves garlic
- 1 cup spinach

DIRECTIONS

Blend the paprika, garlic powder, and salt and sprinkle over both sides of the chicken.

Melt the butter in a frying pan (choose medium heat). Add the chicken breast and fry for 5 minutes each side. Set aside.

Add the heavy cream, sun-dried tomatoes, and garlic to the pan and whisk well to combine. Cook for 2 minutes. Add spinach and sauté for an additional 3 minutes. Return the chicken to the pan and cover with the sauce.

Nutrition: 26g Fat 4g Protein 280 Calories

208. CAULIFLOWER CHEESECAKE

PREPARATION
20 MIN

COOKING
30 MIN

SERVES
6

INGREDIENTS

- 1 head cauliflower
- 2/3 cup sour cream
- 4 oz cream cheese, softened
- 1½ cup cheddar cheese
- 6 pieces bacon
- 1 tsp salt
- ½ tsp black pepper
- ¼ cup green onion
- ¼ tsp garlic powder

DIRECTIONS

Preheat the oven to 350°F.

Boil the cauliflower florets for 5 minutes.

In a separate bowl combine the cream cheese and sour cream. Mix well and add the cheddar cheese, bacon pieces, green onion, salt, pepper, and garlic powder. Put the cauliflower florets into the bowl and combine with the sauce.

Put the cauliflower mix on the baking tray and bake for 15-20 minutes.

Nutrition: 26g Fat 15g Protein 320 Calories

PREPARATION
5 MIN

COOKING
15 MIN

SERVES
4

209. CHINESE PORK BOWL

INGREDIENTS

- 1¼ pounds pork belly
- 2 Tbsp tamari soy sauce
- 1 Tbsp rice vinegar
- 2 cloves garlic, smashed
- 3 oz butter
- 1-pound Brussels sprouts
- ½ leek, chopped

DIRECTIONS

Fry the pork over medium-high heat until it is starting to turn golden brown.

Combine the garlic cloves, butter, and Brussel sprouts. Add to the pan, whisk well and cook until the sprouts turn golden brown.

Stir the soy sauce and rice vinegar together and pour the sauce into the pan.

Sprinkle with salt and pepper.

Top with chopped leek.

Nutrition: 97g Fat 19g Protein 993 Calories

PREPARATION
20 MIN

210. TURKEY-PEPPER MIX

COOKING
0 MIN

SERVES
1

INGREDIENTS

- ▸ 1-pound turkey tenderloin
- ▸ 1 tsp salt, divided
- ▸ 2 Tbsp extra-virgin olive oil
- ▸ ½ sweet onion, sliced
- ▸ 1 red bell pepper, cut into strips
- ▸ 1 yellow bell pepper, cut into strips
- ▸ ½ tsp Italian seasoning
- ▸ ¼ tsp ground black pepper
- ▸ 2 tsp red wine vinegar
- ▸ 1 14-ounces can crush tomatoes

DIRECTIONS

Sprinkle ½ tsp salt on your turkey. Pour 1 Tbsp oil into the pan and heat it. Add the turkey steaks and cook for 1-3 minutes per side. Set aside.

Put the onion, bell peppers, and the remaining salt to the pan and cook for 7 minutes, stirring all the time. Sprinkle with Italian seasoning and add black pepper. Cook for 30 seconds. Add the tomatoes and vinegar and fry the mix for about 20 seconds.

Return the turkey to the pan and pour the sauce over it. Simmer for 2-3 minutes.

Top with chopped parsley and basil.

Nutrition: 8g Fat 30g Protein 230 Calories

PREPARATION
5 MIN

COOKING
10 MIN

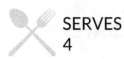

SERVES
4

211. SHRIMP SCAMPI WITH GARLIC

INGREDIENTS

- 1-pound shrimp
- 3 Tbsp olive oil
- 1 bulb shallot, sliced
- 4 cloves garlic, minced
- ½ cup Pinot Grigio
- 4 Tbsp salted butter
- 1 Tbsp lemon juice
- ½ tsp sea salt
- ¼ tsp black pepper
- ¼ tsp red pepper flakes
- ¼ cup parsley, chopped

DIRECTIONS

Pour the olive oil into the previously heated frying pan. Add the garlic and shallots and fry for about 2 minutes.

Combine the Pinot Grigio, salted butter, and lemon juice. Pour this mix into the pan and cook for 5 minutes.

Put the parsley, black pepper, red pepper flakes, and sea salt into the pan and whisk well.

Add the shrimp and fry until they are pink (about 3 minutes).

Nutrition: 7g Fat 32g Protein 344 Calories

PREPARATION
15 MIN

COOKING
15 MIN

SERVES
4

212. PORK CUTLETS WITH SPANISH ONION

INGREDIENTS

- 1 tablespoon olive oil
- 2 pork cutlets
- 1 bell pepper, deveined and sliced
- 1 Spanish onion, chopped
- 2 garlic cloves, minced
- 1/2 teaspoon hot sauce
- 1/2 teaspoon mustard
- 1/2 teaspoon paprika

DIRECTIONS

Fry the pork cutlets for 3 to 4 minutes until evenly golden and crispy on both sides.

Decrease the temperature to medium and add the bell pepper, Spanish onion, garlic, hot sauce, and mustard; continue cooking until the vegetables have softened, for a further 3 minutes.

Sprinkle with paprika, salt, and black pepper. Serve immediately and enjoy!

Nutrition: 403 Calories 24.1g Fat 3.4g Total Carbs

PREPARATION
15 MIN

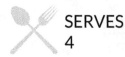

COOKING
15 MIN

SERVES
4

213. RICH AND EASY PORK RAGOUT

INGREDIENTS

- 1 teaspoon lard, melted at room temperature
- 3/4-pound pork butt
- 1 red bell pepper
- 1 poblano pepper
- 2 cloves garlic
- 1/2 cup leeks
- 1/2 teaspoon mustard seeds
- 1/4 teaspoon ground allspice
- 1/4 teaspoon celery seeds
- 1 cup roasted vegetable broth
- 2 vine-ripe tomatoes, pureed

DIRECTIONS

Melt the lard in a stockpot over moderate heat. Once hot, cook the pork cubes for 4 to 6 minutes, occasionally stirring to ensure even cooking.

Then, stir in the vegetables and continue cooking until they are tender and fragrant. Add in the salt, black pepper, mustard seeds, allspice, celery seeds, roasted vegetable broth, and tomatoes.

Reduce the heat to simmer. Let it simmer for 30 minutes longer or until everything is heated through. Ladle into individual bowls and serve hot. Bon appétit!

Nutrition: 389 Calories 24.3g Fat 5.4g Total Carbs

214. MELT-IN-YOUR-MOUTH PORK ROAST

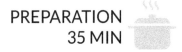

PREPARATION
35 MIN

COOKING
40 MIN

SERVES
2

INGREDIENTS

- 1-pound pork shoulder
- 4 tablespoons red wine
- 1 teaspoon stone-ground mustard
- 1 tablespoon coconut aminos
- 1 tablespoon lemon juice
- 1 tablespoon sesame oil
- 2 sprigs rosemary
- 1 teaspoon sage
- 1shallot, peeled and chopped
- 1/2 celery stalk, chopped

- 1/2 head garlic

DIRECTIONS

Place the pork shoulder, red wine, mustard, coconut aminos, lemon juice, sesame oil, rosemary, and sage in a ceramic dish; cover and let it marinate in your refrigerator at least 1 hour.

Discard a lightly greased baking dish. Scatter the vegetables around the pork shoulder and sprinkle with salt and black pepper. Roast in the preheated oven at 390 degrees F for 15 minutes.

Now, reduce the temperature to 310 degrees F and continue baking an additional 40 to 45 minutes. Baste the meat with the reserved marinade once or twice.

Place on cooling racks before carving and serving. Bon appétit!

Nutrition: 497 Calories 35.3g Fat 40.2g Protein

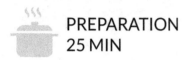

PREPARATION
25 MIN

COOKING
30 MIN

SERVES
2

215. CHUNKY PORK SOUP WITH MUSTARD GREENS

INGREDIENTS

- 1 tablespoon olive oil
- 1 bell pepper, deveined and chopped
- 2 garlic cloves, pressed
- 1/2 cup scallions, chopped
- 1/2-pound ground pork (84% lean)
- 1 cup beef bone broth
- 1 cup of water
- 1/2 teaspoon crushed red pepper flakes
- 1 bay laurel
- 1 teaspoon fish sauce
- 2 cups mustard greens, torn into pieces
- 1 tablespoon fresh parsley, chopped

DIRECTIONS

Coat, once hot, sauté the pepper, garlic, and scallions until tender or about 3 minutes.

After that, stir in the ground pork and cook for 5 minutes more or until well browned, stirring periodically.

Add in the beef bone broth, water, red pepper, salt, black pepper, and bay laurel. Reduce the temperature to simmer and cook, covered, for 10 minutes. Afterward, stir in the fish sauce and mustard greens.

Remove from the heat; let it stand until the greens are wilted. Ladle into individual bowls and serve garnished with fresh parsley.

Nutrition: 344 Calories 25.2g Fat 23.1g Protein

216. PULLED PORK WITH MINT AND CHEESE

PREPARATION
20 MIN

COOKING
15 MIN

SERVES
2

INGREDIENTS

- 1 teaspoon lard, melted at room temperature
- 3/4 pork Boston butt, sliced
- 2 garlic cloves, pressed
- 1/2 teaspoon red pepper flakes, crushed
- 1/2 teaspoon black peppercorns, freshly cracked
- Sea salt, to taste
- 2 bell peppers, deveined and sliced
- 1 tablespoon fresh mint leave snipped

- 4 tablespoons cream cheese

DIRECTIONS

Melt the lard in a cast-iron skillet over a moderate flame. Once hot, brown the pork for 2 minutes per side until caramelized and crispy on the edges.

Reduce the temperature to medium-low and continue cooking another 4 minutes, turning over periodically. Shred the pork with two forks and return to the skillet.

Add the garlic, red pepper, black peppercorns, salt, and bell pepper and continue cooking for a further 2 minutes or until the peppers are just tender and fragrant.

Serve with fresh mint and a dollop of cream cheese. Enjoy!

Nutrition: 370 Calories 21.9g Fat 34.9g Protein

PREPARATION
3 MIN

COOKING
11 MIN

SERVES
1

217. LITTLE PORTOBELLO PIZZA

INGREDIENTS

- 1½ oz. Monterey jack
- 9 spinach leaves
- 3 Portobello mushrooms
- 1½ oz. cheddar cheese
- Olive oil
- 1½ oz. mozzarella
- 12 pepperoni slices
- 3 tomato slices
- 3 tsp. pizza seasoning

DIRECTIONS

Through cleaning them and cutting the gills and the stalks, dress the Portobello mushrooms.

Sprinkle with the seasoning of olive oil and bread, and add the other ingredients, except the pepperoni. Cook 6 minutes at 450 ° F. Add the slices of pepperoni and grill until crumbly.

Nutrition: 409 Calories 20g Fat 31g Protein

218. DUCK AND EGGPLANT CASSEROLE

PREPARATION

+

COOKING
45 MIN

SERVES
4

INGREDIENTS

- 1-pound ground duck meat
- 1 ½ tablespoons ghee, melted
- 1/3 cup double cream
- 1/2-pound eggplant, peeled and sliced
- 1 ½ cups almond flour
- Salt and black pepper, to taste
- 1/2 teaspoon fennel seeds
- 1/2 teaspoon oregano, dried
- 8 eggs

DIRECTIONS

Incorporate almond flour with salt, black, fennel seeds, and oregano. Scourge one egg and the melted ghee.

Pound crust into the bottom of a greased pie pan. Cook the ground duck for 3 minutes.

Scourge rest of eggs and double cream. Mix in the browned meat until well incorporated. Fill mixture into the prepared crust. Garnish with the eggplant slices.

Bake for 40 minutes. Cut into four pieces.

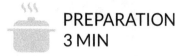

PREPARATION
3 MIN

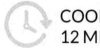

COOKING
12 MIN

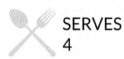

SERVES
4

219. SPICY BREAKFAST SAUSAGE

INGREDIENTS

- ▸ 4 chicken sausages, sliced
- ▸ 1 chili pepper, minced
- ▸ cup shallots, diced
- ▸ 1/4 cup dry white wine
- ▸ teaspoons lard, room temperature
- ▸ teaspoon garlic, minced
- ▸ Spanish peppers, deveined and chopped
- ▸ 2 tablespoons fresh coriander, minced
- ▸ 2 teaspoons balsamic vinegar
- ▸ 1 cup pureed tomatoes

DIRECTIONS

In a frying pan, warm the lard over a moderately high flame.

Then, sear the sausage until well browned on all sides; add in the remaining ingredients and stir to combine.

Allow it to simmer over low heat for 10 minutes or until thickened slightly.

Nutrition: 381 Calories 18g Fat 25g Protein

220. CLASSIC CHICKEN SALAD

PREPARATION
12 MIN

COOKING
8 MIN

SERVES
4

INGREDIENTS

- 1 medium shallot, thinly sliced
- 1 tablespoon Dijon mustard
- tablespoon fresh oregano, chopped
- 1/2 cup mayonnaise
- cups boneless rotisserie chicken, shredded
- 2 avocados
- 3 hard-boiled eggs, cut into quarters

DIRECTIONS

Toss the chicken with the avocado, shallots, and oregano.

Add in the mayonnaise, mustard, salt, and black pepper; stir to combine.

Nutrition: 411 Calories 16g Fat 31g Protein

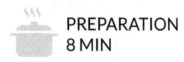

**PREPARATION
8 MIN**

**COOKING
11 MIN**

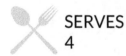

**SERVES
4**

221. CREAMED SAUSAGE WITH SPAGHETTI SQUASH

INGREDIENTS

- 1 ½ pound cheese & bacon chicken sausages, sliced
- 8 ounces' spaghetti squash
- 1/2 cup green onions, finely chopped
- 2/3 cup double cream
- 1 Spanish pepper, deveined and finely minced
- garlic clove, pressed
- teaspoons butter, room temperature
- 1 ¼ cups cream of onion soup

DIRECTIONS

Cook butter in saucepan at moderate flame. Then, sear the sausages until no longer pink about 9 minutes. Reserve.

In the same saucepan, cook the green onions, pepper, and garlic until they've softened.

Add in the spaghetti squash, salt, black pepper and cream of onion soup; bring to a boil.

Reduce the heat to medium-low and fold in the cream; let it simmer until the sauce has reduced slightly or about 7 minutes. Add in the reserved sausage and gently stir to combine.

Nutrition: 401 Calories 16g Fat 32g Protein

222. CHICKEN FAJITAS WITH PEPPERS AND CHEESE

PREPARATION 8 MIN

COOKING 6 MIN

SERVES 4

INGREDIENTS

- 1 Habanero pepper
- 4 banana peppers
- 1 teaspoon Mexican seasoning blend
- 2 garlic cloves, minced
- 1 cup onions, chopped
- 1-pound chicken, ground
- 1/3 cup dry sherry
- 1/2 cup Coria cheese, shredded

DIRECTIONS

In a pan, cook avocado oil over medium heat.

Sauté the garlic, onions, and peppers until they are tender and aromatic or about 5 minutes.

Fold in the ground chicken and continue to cook until the juices run clear.

Add in the dry sherry, Mexican seasonings, salt, and pepper.

Cook for additional 6 minutes.

Nutrition: 391 Calories 10g Fat 29g Protein

PREPARATION
18 MIN

COOKING
32 MIN

SERVES
4

223. CRISPY CHICKEN DRUMSTICKS

INGREDIENTS

- 4 chicken drumsticks
- 1/4 tsp. black pepper
- 1 teaspoon dried basil
- 1 teaspoon dried oregano
- 1 tablespoon olive oil
- 1 teaspoon paprika

DIRECTIONS

Pat dry the chicken drumsticks and rub them with olive oil, salt, black pepper, paprika, basil, and oregano.

Preheat your oven to 410 degrees F. Coat a baking pan with a piece of parchment paper.

Bake the chicken drumsticks until they are browned on all sides for 40 to 45 minutes.

Nutrition: 408 Calories 18g Fat 28g Protein

224. CHICKEN FILLET WITH BRUSSELS SPROUTS

PREPARATION
8 MIN

COOKING
11 MIN

SERVES
4

INGREDIENTS

- 3/4-pound chicken breasts
- 1/2 teaspoon ancho Chile powder
- 1/2 teaspoon whole black peppercorns
- 1/2 cup onions, chopped
- cup vegetable broth
- tablespoons olive oil
- 1 ½ lb. Brussels sprouts
- 1/4 teaspoon garlic salt
- clove garlic, minced
- tablespoons port wine

DIRECTIONS

Heat 1 tablespoon of oil in frying pan over medium-high heat. Sauté the Brussels sprouts for about 3 minutes or until golden on all sides. Salt to taste and reserve.

Heat the remaining tablespoon of olive oil—Cook the garlic and chicken for about 3 minutes.

Add in the onions, vegetable broth, wine, Ancho Chile powder, and black peppercorns; bring to a boil. Then, reduce the temperature to simmer and continue to cook for 4 to 5 minutes longer.

Add the reserved Brussels sprouts back to the frying pan.

Nutrition: 399 Calories 12g Fat 33g Protein

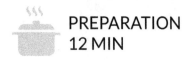

PREPARATION
12 MIN

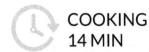

COOKING
14 MIN

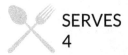

SERVES
4

225. CHICKEN BREASTS WITH MUSTARD SAUCE

INGREDIENTS

- 1/4 cup vegetable broth
- Salt and pepper, to taste
- 1/2 cup fresh parsley,
- 1/2 cup heavy whipped cream
- 1/2 cup onions, chopped
- 2 garlic cloves, minced
- 1/4 cup Marsala wine
- 2 tablespoons brown mustard
- 1 tablespoon olive oil
- 1-pound chicken breasts, butterflied

DIRECTIONS

Preheat oil in frying pan at moderate flame. Cook chicken breasts for about 6 minutes; season with salt and pepper to taste and reserve.

Cook the onion and garlic until it is fragrant or about 5 minutes. Add in the wine to scrape the bits that may be stuck to the bottom of your frying pan.

Boil broth. Fold in the double cream, mustard, and parsley.

Nutrition: 402 Calories 15g Fat 29g Protein

226. CHINESE-STYLE CABBAGE WITH TURKEY

PREPARATION
22 MIN

COOKING
24 MIN

SERVES
4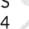

INGREDIENTS

- ▸ pound turkey, ground
- ▸ slices smoked bacon, chopped
- ▸ 1-pound Chinese cabbage, finely chopped
- ▸ 1 tablespoon sesame oil
- ▸ 1/2 cup onions, chopped
- ▸ teaspoon ginger-garlic paste
- ▸ ripe tomatoes, chopped
- ▸ 1 teaspoon Five-spice powder

DIRECTIONS

Preheat oil in wok over a moderate flame. Cook the onions until tender and translucent.

Now, add in the remaining ingredients and bring to a boil. Reduce the temperature to medium-low and partially cover.

Reduce the heat to medium-low and cook an additional 30 minutes, crumbling the turkey and bacon with a fork.

Nutrition: 399 Calories 17g Fat 34g Protein

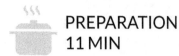

PREPARATION
11 MIN

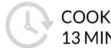

COOKING
13 MIN

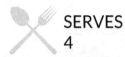

SERVES
4

227. EASY TURKEY MEATBALLS

INGREDIENTS

- **For Meatballs:**
- 1/3 cup Colby cheese, freshly grated
- 3/4-pound ground turkey
- 1/3 teaspoon Five-spice powder
- 1 egg
- **For Sauce:**
- 1/3 cups water
- 1/3 cup champagne vinegar
- tablespoons soy sauce
- 1/2 cup Swerve
- 1/2 cup tomato sauces
- 1/2 tsp. paprika

- 1/3 tsp. guar gum

DIRECTIONS

Thoroughly combine all ingredients for the meatballs. Roll the mixture into balls and sear them until browned on all sides.

In a saucepan, mix all of the sauce ingredients and cook until the sauce has thickened, whisking continuously.

Fold the meatballs into the sauce and continue to cook, partially covered, for about 10 minutes.

Nutrition: 408 Calories 19g Fat 35g Protein

228. CHICKEN WITH MEDITERRANEAN SAUCE

PREPARATION 4 MIN

COOKING 16 MIN

SERVES 6

INGREDIENTS

- ▶ 1 stick butter
- ▶ ½ pounds of chicken breasts
- ▶ teaspoons red wine vinegar
- ▶ ½ tablespoons olive oil
- ▶ 1/3 cup fresh Italian parsley, chopped
- ▶ tablespoon green garlic
- ▶ 2 tablespoons red onions
- ▶ Flaky sea salt and ground black pepper, to taste

DIRECTIONS

In a cast-iron skillet, heat the oil over a moderate flame. Sear the chicken for 10 to 12 minutes or until no longer pink. Season with salt and black pepper.

Add in the melted butter and continue to cook until heated through. Stir in the green garlic, onion, and Italian parsley; let it cook for 3 to 4 minutes more.

Mix in red wine vinegar and pull away from the heat.

Nutrition: 411 Calories 21g Fat 36g Protein

PREPARATION
1 H

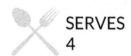

COOKING
40 MIN

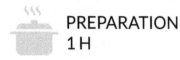

SERVES
4

229. EASY ROASTED TURKEY DRUMSTICKS

INGREDIENTS

- 2 turkey drumsticks
- 1 ½ tablespoon sesame oil
- 1 tablespoon poultry seasoning
- **For the Sauce:**
- 1-ounce Cottage cheese
- 1-ounce full-fat sour cream
- small-sized avocado, pitted and mashed
- tablespoons fresh parsley, finely chopped
- 1 teaspoon fresh lemon juice
- 1/3 teaspoon sea salt

DIRECTIONS

Pat the turkey drumsticks dry and sprinkle them with the poultry seasoning.

Brush a baking pan with the sesame oil.

Place the turkey drumsticks on the baking pan.

Roast in the preheated oven at 350 degrees F for about 1 hour 30 minutes, rotating the pan halfway through the cooking time.

In the meantime, make the sauce by whisking all the sauce ingredients.

Nutrition: 415 Calories 12g Fat 26g Protein

PREPARATION
18 MIN

230. HERBED CHICKEN BREASTS

COOKING
24 MIN

SERVES
8

INGREDIENTS

- ▶ 4 chicken breasts
- ▶ 1 Italian pepper
- ▶ 10 black olives, pitted
- ▶ ½ cups vegetable broth
- ▶ garlic cloves, pressed
- ▶ 2 tablespoons olive oil
- ▶ 1 tablespoon Old Sub Sailor

DIRECTIONS

Rub the chicken with the garlic and Old Sub Sailor; salt to taste. Heat the oil in a frying pan over moderately high heat.

Sear the chicken until it is browned on all sides, about 5 minutes.

Add in the pepper, olives, and vegetable broth and bring it to boil. Decrease heat to simmer and cook, partially covered, for extra 35 minutes.

Nutrition: 397 Calories 17g Fat 35g Protein

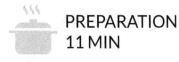

231. CHEESE AND PROSCIUTTO CHICKEN ROULADE

PREPARATION
11 MIN

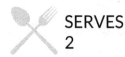

COOKING
26 MIN

SERVES
2

INGREDIENTS

- 1/2 cup Ricotta cheese
- 4 slices of prosciutto
- 1-pound chicken fillet
- 1 tablespoon fresh coriander
- 1 teaspoon cayenne pepper

DIRECTIONS

Season the chicken fillet with salt and pepper. Spread the Ricotta cheese over the chicken fillet; sprinkle with the fresh coriander.

Roll up and cut into 4 pieces. Wrap each piece with one slice of prosciutto; secure with kitchen twine.

Place the wrapped chicken in a parchment-lined baking pan. Now, bake in the preheated oven at 385 degrees F for about 30 minutes.

Nutrition: 408 Calories 20g Fat 34g Protein

CHAPTER 9. DESSERT RECIPES

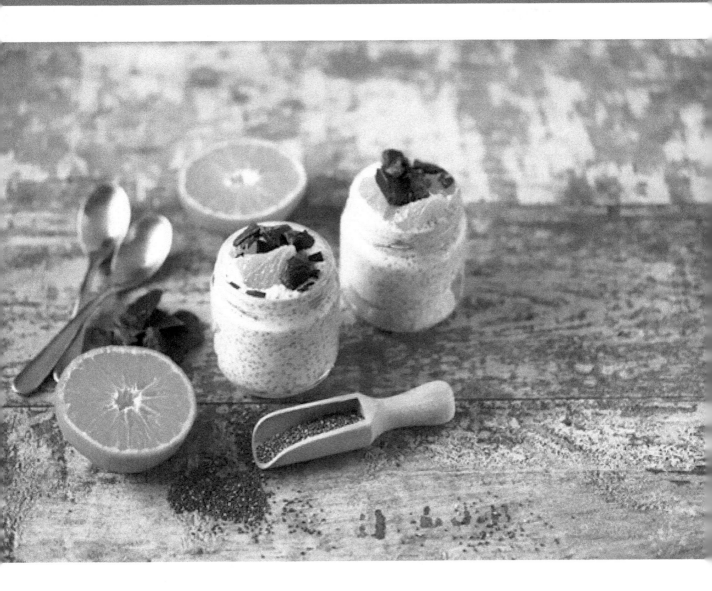

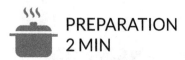

PREPARATION
2 MIN

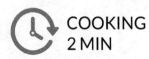

COOKING
2 MIN

SERVES
2

232. CHOCOLATE MUG MUFFIN

INGREDIENTS

- 2 tbsp almond four
- 1 tbsp cocoa powder
- 1 tbsp Swerve
- ½ tsp baking powder
- ¼ tsp vanilla extract
- 1 egg
- 1 pinch sea salt
- 1 ½ tbsp melted coconut oil or butter
- ½ ounce sugar-free dark chocolate
- ½ tsp coconut oil or butter for greasing the mugs

DIRECTIONS

Combine dry ingredients in a small bowl. Stir in egg and melted coconut oil or butter. Mix until smooth.

Add coarsely chopped chocolate and pour into two well-greased coffee mugs.

Microwave for 90 seconds. Remove and let cool

Serve with a dollop of whipped coconut cream.

Nutrition: 230 Calories 6g Protein 21g Fat

233. LOW CARB CHOCOLATE MOUSSE

PREPARATION
2 MIN
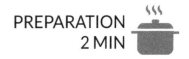

COOKING
15 MIN
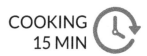

SERVES
6
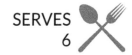

INGREDIENTS

- 1 ¼ cups heavy whipping cream
- ½ tsp vanilla extract
- 2 egg yolks
- 1 pinch sea salt
- 3 ounces dark chocolate with a minimum of 80% cocoa solids

DIRECTIONS

Break or chop the chocolate into small pieces. Melt in the microwave (20 second intervals, stirring in between). Set aside at room temperature to cool.

Whip the cream to soft peaks. Add vanilla towards the end.

Mix egg yolks with salt in a separate bowl.

Add the melted chocolate to the egg yolks and mix to a smooth batter.

Add a couple of spoonsful of whipped cream to the chocolate mix and stir to loosen it a bit. Add the remaining cream and fold it through.

Divide the batter into ramekins or serving glasses of your choice. Place in the fridge and let chill for at least 2 hours. Serve as is, or top with fresh berries.

Nutrition: 270 Calories 3g Protein 25g Fat

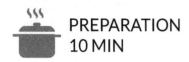

PREPARATION
10 MIN

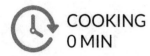

COOKING
0 MIN

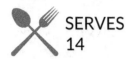

SERVES
14

234. STRAWBERRY CHEESECAKE FAT BOMBS

INGREDIENTS

- ½ cup strawberries
- ¾ cup cream cheese, softened
- ¼ cup butter
- 2 tbsp powdered erythritol
- ½ teaspoon vanilla extract

· ·

DIRECTIONS

Place the cream cheese and butter (cut into small pieces) into a mixing bowl. Leave at room temperature for 30 -60 minutes.

Meanwhile, wash the strawberries and remove the green parts. Place the in a bowl and mash, using a fork or place in a blender for a smooth texture.

Add the powdered erythritol, vanilla extract and mix well. Before you mix the strawberries with the remaining ingredients, make sure they have reached room temperature.

Add to the bowl with the softened butter and cream cheese.

Use a hand whisk or food processor and mix until well combined.

Spoon the mixture into small muffin silicon molds, or candy molds. Place in the freezer for about 2 hours or until set.

When done, unmold the fat bombs and place into a container. Keep in the freezer and enjoy any time.

Nutrition: 67 Calories 0.9g Protein 7.4g Fat

235. CHOCOLATE CHIP COOKIE DOUGH FAT BOMBS

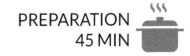

PREPARATION
45 MIN

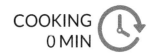

COOKING
0 MIN

SERVES
6

INGREDIENTS

- ► 8 ounces cream cheese, softened
- ► 1 stick (1/2 cup) salted butter
- ► ½ cup creamy peanut butter or almond butter
- ► 1/3 cup swerve sweetener
- ► 1 tsp vanilla extract
- ► 4 ounces Stevia sweetened chocolate chips

DIRECTIONS

Cream everything together in a mixer and then spray a cookie scoop with coconut oil cooking spray.

Refrigerate dough for 30 minutes before scooping onto parchment paper, then freeze for 30 minutes.

Store in refrigerator.

Nutrition: 139 Calories 2g Protein 14g Fat

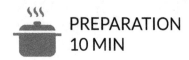

PREPARATION
10 MIN

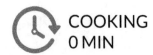

COOKING
0 MIN

SERVES
4

236. NO BAKE KETO MOCHA CHEESECAKE

INGREDIENTS

- ¾ cup heavy whipping cream
- 1 block of cream cheese (room temperature)
- ¼ cup unsweetened cocoa
- ¾ cup Swerve Confectioners sweetener
- 1 double shot of espresso

DIRECTIONS

Place the softened cream cheese in a bowl, and using a hand mixer, whip the cream cheese for 1 minute. Add espresso and continue mixing.

Add the sweetener, ¼ cup at a time and mix. Be sure to taste periodically, you may not need to use all the sweetener.

Add cocoa powder and mix until completely blended.

In a separate bowl, whip the cream until stiff peaks form.

Gently fold the whipped cream into the mocha mixture using a spatula.

Place in individual serving dishes. Enjoy!

Nutrition: 425 Calories 6g Protein 33g Fat

PREPARATION 10 MIN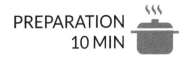

COOKING 10 MIN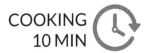

SERVES 24

237. KETO CREAM CHEESE COOKIES

INGREDIENTS

- ¼ cup butter (softened)
- 2 ounces plain cream cheese (softened)
- ½ cup erythritol
- 2 tsp vanilla extract
- 3 cups almond flour
- ¼ tsp sea salt
- 1 large egg white

DIRECTIONS

Preheat oven to 350°F. Line a large cookie sheet with parchment paper.

Use a hand mixer to beat together the butter, cream cheese, and erythritol: beat until fluffy and light in color.

Beat in the vanilla extract, salt and egg white.

Beat in almond flour, ½ cup at a time.

Use a medium cookie scoop to scoop balls of dough onto the prepared cookie sheet. Flatten with your palm.

Bake for 15 minutes, until the edges are lightly golden. Allow to cool completely in the pan before handling (cookies will harden as they cool).

Nutrition: 106 Calories 3g Protein 9g Fat

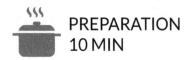

PREPARATION
10 MIN

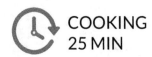

COOKING
25 MIN

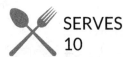

SERVES
10

238. KETO AVOCADO BROWNIES

INGREDIENTS

- ½ cup avocado, mashed
- ½ cup almond butter
- 3 tbsp artificial sweetener
- 2 tbsp cocoa powder
- 1 tbsp olive oil
- 1 tsp vanilla extract
- ½ cup dark chocolate baking chips
- ¼ cup chopped pecans (optional)

DIRECTIONS

Preheat oven to 350°F.

Mash 1 to 1 ½ avocados until you have ½ cup of well mashed avocado.

Using a medium sized mixing bowl, add the mashed avocado and almond butter, beat on high for 2 minutes or until the mixture is creamy and smooth.

Mix in sweetener and cocoa powder. Blend until ingredients are well combined.

Add olive oil and vanilla extract. Stir well until mixture is smooth.

Fold in baking chips and chopped pecans.

Spread the mixture into a well-greased 8x8 baking pan.

Bake for 20 – 25 minutes. Let the brownies cool for at least 10 minutes before you serve.

Nutrition: 680 Calories 9g Protein 13g Fat

239. LOW CARB BUTTER COOKIES

PREPARATION
10 MIN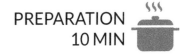

COOKING
10 MIN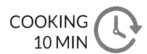

SERVES
6

INGREDIENTS

- ► 1 cup almond flour
- ► ¼ cup Confectioners Swerve
- ► 3 tbsp salted butter (room temperature)
- ► ½ tsp vanilla extract

• •

DIRECTIONS

Preheat oven to 350°F.

Prepare a baking sheet lined with parchment paper or a nonstick baking mat.

In a mixing bowl, combine all ingredients, stirring thoroughly until resembling a dough. (it will look crumbly while you stir, then will form into a cohesive dough)

Form 1-inch balls, placing them on the baking sheet. There should be about 12 balls, separated from each other by about 2 inches.

Flatten each dough ball using a fork, then rotate 90 degrees and flatten again, forming a crisscross pattern.

Bake at 350°F until the cookie are golden around the edges, 8-10 minutes depending on the thickness of the cookies.

Let cool completely before removing them from the baking sheet, they cookies will be very soft when they first come out of the oven.

Nutrition: 80 Calories 2g Protein 8g Fat

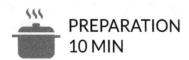

PREPARATION
10 MIN

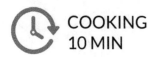

COOKING
10 MIN

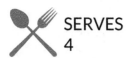

SERVES
4

240. AVOCADO FROZEN YOGURT

INGREDIENTS

- 2 ½ cups whipping cream (sugar-free)
- 1 cup Greek yogurt
- 1 tbsp cherry extract (sugar-free)
- 1 tsp Stevia powder
- 1 tbsp arrowroot powder
- ½ avocado, cut into chunks
- 1-ounce gelatin

DIRECTIONS

In a large mixing bowl combine Greek yogurt, cherry extract, stevia and arrowroot powder and 2 cups whipping cream. With an electric mixer, blend for 2-3 minutes on high speed. Pour the mixture into serving glasses and place in freezer for 30-40 minutes.

Boil the gelatin with a cup of water. Stir well to dissolve the gelatin completely. When done, remove from the heat and allow the gelatin to cool to room temperature.

Chop the avocado into bite-sized pieces after slicing them in half and peeling off the skin. Set aside.

Add 2 tablespoons of gelatin on top of the frozen yogurt. Put some avocado chunks as well. Put in the rest of the whipping cream and replace in the freezer for another 15 minutes.

Serve cold.

Nutrition: 285 Calories 13g Protein 24g Fat

241. BLUEBERRY MUG CAKE

PREPARATION
3 MIN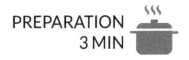

COOKING
2 MIN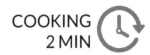

SERVES
2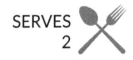

INGREDIENTS

- 2 tbsp coconut flour
- ½ tsp baking powder
- 25 grams fresh blueberries
- 1 large egg
- 2 tbsp cream cheese
- 1 tbsp butter
- 15 – 20 drips Liquid Stevia
- ¼ tsp Himalayan Salt

DIRECTIONS

Add the butter and cream cheese to a mug and microwave for 20 seconds. Mix with a fork.

Add the baking powder, coconut flour and stevia and combine with a fork.

Add the egg and combine.

Add the salt and fresh blueberries, and fold gently.

Microwave for 90 seconds.

Eat right out of the mug, or flip out onto a plate. For added flavor dust with powdered swerve.

Nutrition: 345 Calories 10g Protein 29g Fat

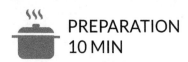

PREPARATION
10 MIN

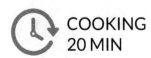

COOKING
20 MIN

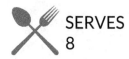

SERVES
8

242. RICOTTA GELATO

INGREDIENTS

- 2 cups fresh cheese
- 2 cups unsweetened almond milk
- 1/8 teaspoon ground cinnamon
- 1/8 teaspoon ground nutmeg
- 1 cup Erythritol
- 5 large organic egg yolk
- 1 cup heavy cream

DIRECTIONS

Line a sieve with a cheesecloth and arrange over a bowl.

Place the ricotta cheese in sieve.

Refrigerate the bowl of ricotta cheese overnight to drain.

In a medium pan, mix together the almond milk, cinnamon, and nutmeg over medium-low heat and bring to a gentle simmer.

Remove the pan from the heat and set aside.

In a bowl, add the Erythritol and egg yolks and with an electric mixer, beat on high speed until thick and pale yellow.

Add ½ of the warm milk mixture and beat until well combined.

Transfer the mixture into the pan with remaining milk mixture.

Return the pan over low heat and cook until mixture becomes thick, stirring continuously.

Remove the pan from heat and immediately, stir in the heavy cream.

Arrange a fine sieve over a bowl.

Strain the milk mixture in the bowl and cool over ice bath.

Now, with the electric mixer, beat the mixture completely.

Transfer the mixture into an ice cream maker and freeze according to manufacturer's directions.

Now, transfer the mixture into sealable container and freeze until set completely before serving.

Nutrition: 181 Calories 14.2g Fat 9.3g Protein

PREPARATION
10 MIN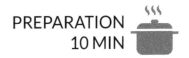

COOKING
0 MIN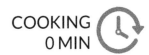

SERVES
4

243. LEMON MOUSSE

INGREDIENTS

- ¼ cup fresh lemon juice
- 8 ounces cream cheese, softened
- 1 cup heavy cream
- 1/8 teaspoon salt
- ½-1 teaspoon lemon liquid stevia

DIRECTIONS

Put the lemon juice and cream cheese in a blender, and pulse until smooth.

Add remaining ingredients and pulse until well combined and fluffy.

Transfer the mixture into serving glasses and refrigerate to chill before serving.

Nutrition: 305 Calories 32g Fat 9.3g Protein

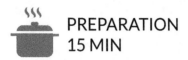

PREPARATION
15 MIN

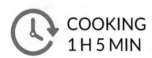

COOKING
1 H 5 MIN

SERVES
8

244. CREAM CHEESE FLAN

INGREDIENTS

- ¾ cup granulated Erythritol, divided
- 3 tablespoons water, divided
- 2 teaspoons organic vanilla extract, divided
- 5 large organic eggs
- 2 cups heavy whipping cream
- 8 ounces full-fat cream cheese, softened
- ¼ teaspoon sea salt

DIRECTIONS

Preheat the oven to 3500F.

Grease an 8-inch cake pan.

For caramel: In a heavy-bottomed pan, add ½ cup of the Erythritol, 2 tablespoons of water, and 1 teaspoon of vanilla extract over medium-low heat and cook until sweetener is melted completely, stirring continuously.

Remove from the heat and place the caramel in the bottom of the prepared cake pan evenly.

In a blender, add the remaining Erythritol, vanilla extract, heavy cream, cream cheese, eggs, and salt, and pulse until smooth.

Place the cream cheese mixture over caramel evenly.

Arrange the cake pan into a large roasting pan.

In the roasting pan, add the hot water about 1-inch up sides of the cake pan.

Place the roasting pan in oven and bake for approximately 1 hour or until center becomes set.

Remove from the oven and place the cake pan in water bath to cool completely.

Refrigerate for about 4–5 hours before serving.

Nutrition: 250 Calories 24g Fat 6.7g Protein

PREPARATION
10 MIN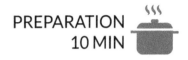

COOKING
5 MIN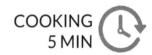

SERVES
4

245. VANILLA PANNA COTTA

INGREDIENTS

- 2 teaspoons unflavored gelatin powder
- 2 tablespoons water
- 2 cups heavy whipping cream
- 1 tablespoon organic vanilla extract
- 4 tablespoons fresh raspberries

DIRECTIONS

In a bowl, add the gelatin and water and mix until well combined. Set aside.

In a pan, add cream and vanilla extract and bring to a boil.

Set the heat to medium-low and simmer for about 2 minutes.

Remove the pan of cream from heat and mix in the gelatin mixture until well combined.

Transfer the mixture into serving glasses evenly and set aside to cool completely.

With a plastic wrap, cover each glass and refrigerate for about 4–5 hours.

Remove the glasses from refrigerator and set aside at room temperature for about 30 minutes before serving.

Serve with the garnishing of raspberries.

Nutrition: 226 Calories 22g Fat 2.7g Protein

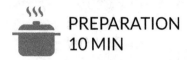 **PREPARATION**
10 MIN

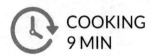 **COOKING**
9 MIN

 **SERVES**
2

246. LAVA CAKE

INGREDIENTS

- 2 ounces unsweetened dark chocolate
- 2 ounces unsalted butter
- 2 organic eggs
- 2 tablespoons powdered Erythritol
- 1 tablespoon almond flour

DIRECTIONS

Preheat the oven to 3500F.

Grease 2 ramekins.

In a microwave-safe bowl, add the chocolate and butter and microwave on High for about 2 minutes, stirring after every 30 seconds.

Remove from the microwave and stir until smooth.

Place the eggs in a bowl and with a wire whisk, beat well.

Add the chocolate mixture, Erythritol, and almond flour, and mix until well combined.

Divide the mixture into the prepared ramekins evenly.

Bake for approximately 9 minutes or until the top is set.

Remove the ramekins from oven and set aside for about 1–2 minutes.

Carefully, invert the cakes onto the serving plates and dust with extra powdered Erythritol.

Nutrition: 478 Calories 44g Fat 9.6g Protein

PREPARATION
20 MIN

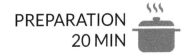

247. LIME PIE

COOKING
20 MIN

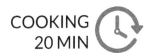

SERVES
8

INGREDIENTS

- **Crust**
- ½ cup almond flour
- ½ cup coconut flour, sifted
- ¼ cup granulated Erythritol
- ¼ cup unsalted butter, melted
- 2 organic eggs
- ¼ teaspoon salt
- **Filling**
- ¾ cup unsweetened coconut milk
- ½ cup granulated Erythritol

- ¼ cup heavy cream
- 2 teaspoons xanthan gum
- 1 teaspoon guar gum
- ¼ teaspoon powdered stevia
- 3 organic egg yolks
- ½ cup fresh key lime juice
- 2 tablespoons unsweetened dried coconut
- **Topping**
- 1 cup whipped cream
- ½ key lime, cut into slices

DIRECTIONS

Preheat your oven to 4000F.

For crust: Add all ingredients in a bowl and mix until well combined.

With your hands, knead the dough for about 1 minute.

Make a ball from the dough.

Arrange the dough ball between 2 sheets of wax paper and with a rolling pin, roll into 1/8-inch thick circle.

In a 9-inch pie dish, place the dough and with your hands, press the mixture in the bottom and up sides.

Now, with a fork, prick the bottom and sides of crust at many places.

Bake for approximately 10 minutes.

Remove from the oven and place the crust onto a wire rack to cool.

Now, set the temperature of oven to 3500F (1800C).

For filling: In a food processor, add the coconut milk, Erythritol, heavy cream, xanthan gum, guar gum, and stevia, and pulse until well combined.

Add the egg yolks and lime juice and pulse until well combined.

Place the filling mixture over the crust and with the back of a spoon, spread evenly.

Bake for approximately 10 minutes.

Remove from the oven and place the pie dish onto a wire rack to cool for about 10 minutes.

Now, freeze the pie for about 3–4 hours before serving.

Remove from the freezer and garnish the pie with the whipped cream and lemon slices.

Cut into desired-sized slices and serve.

Nutrition: 251 Calories 24g Fat 5.1g Protein

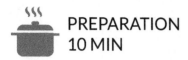

PREPARATION
10 MIN

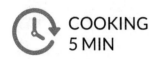

COOKING
5 MIN

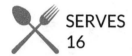

SERVES
16

248. PEANUT BUTTER FUDGE

INGREDIENTS

- 1½ cups creamy, salted peanut butter
- 1/3 cup butter
- 2/3 cup powdered Erythritol
- ¼ cup unsweetened protein powder
- 1 teaspoon organic vanilla extract

DIRECTIONS

In a small pan, add peanut butter and butter over low heat and cook until melted and smooth.

Add the Erythritol and protein powder and mix until smooth.

Remove from the heat and stir in vanilla extract.

Place the fudge mixture onto baking paper-lined 8x8-inch baking dish evenly and with a spatula, smooth the top surface.

Freeze for about 30–45 minutes or until set completely.

Carefully, transfer the fudge onto a cutting board with the help of the parchment paper.

Cut the fudge into equal sized squares and serve.

Nutrition: 184 Calories 16g Fat 10g Protein

249. MASCARPONE BROWNIES

PREPARATION
16 MIN
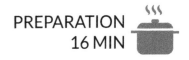

COOKING
28 MIN
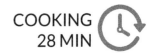

SERVES
16

INGREDIENTS

- ▸ 5 ounces unsweetened dark chocolate
- ▸ 4 tablespoons unsalted butter
- ▸ 3 large organic eggs
- ▸ ½ cup Erythritol
- ▸ ¼ cup mascarpone cheese
- ▸ ¼ cup cacao powder, divided
- ▸ ½ teaspoon salt

DIRECTIONS

Preheat the oven to 3750F.

Line a 9x9-inch baking sheet with a parchment paper.

In a medium microwave-safe bowl, add the chocolate and microwave on High for about 2 minutes or until melted completely, stirring after every 30 seconds.

Add the butter and microwave for about 1 minute or until melted and smooth, stirring once after every 10 seconds.

Remove from the microwave and stir until smooth.

Set aside to cool slightly.

In a large bowl, add the eggs and Erythritol and with an electric mixer, beat on high speed until frothy.

Add the mascarpone cheese and beat until smooth.

Add 2 tablespoons of the cacao powder and salt and gently stir to combine.

Now, sift in the remaining cacao powder and stir until well combined.

Add the melted chocolate mixture into the egg mixture and mix well until well combined.

Place the mixture into the prepared pan evenly.

Bake for approximately 25 minutes.

Remove from the oven and let it cool completely before cutting.

With a sharp knife, cut into desired sized squares and serve.

Nutrition: 93 Calories 9.2g Fat 3g Protein

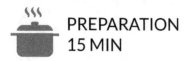
PREPARATION
15 MIN

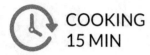
COOKING
15 MIN

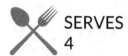
SERVES
4

250. ZUCCHINI MUFFINS

INGREDIENTS

- 4 organic eggs
- ¼ cup unsalted butter, melted
- ¼ cup water
- 1/3 cup coconut flour
- ½ teaspoon organic baking powder
- ¼ teaspoon salt
- 1½ cups zucchini, grated
- ½ cup Parmesan cheese, shredded
- 1 tablespoon fresh oregano, minced
- 1 tablespoon fresh thyme, minced
- ¼ cup cheddar cheese, grated

DIRECTIONS

Preheat the oven to 400°F.

Lightly, grease 8 muffin tins.

Add eggs, butter, and water in a mixing bowl and beat until well combined.

Add the flour, baking powder, and salt, and mix well.

Add remaining ingredients except for cheddar and mix until just combined.

Place the mixture into prepared muffin cups evenly.

Bake for approximately 13–15 minutes or until top of muffins become golden-brown.

Remove the muffin tin from oven and situate onto a wire rack for 10 minutes.

Carefully invert the muffins onto a platter and serve warm.

Nutrition: 287 Calories 23g Fat 13.2g Protein

PREPARATION
15 MIN

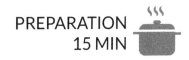

251. LEMON POPPY SEED MUFFINS

COOKING
20 MIN

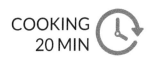

SERVES
6

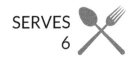

INGREDIENTS

- ¾ cup blanched almond flour
- ¼ cup golden flax meal
- 1/3 cup Erythritol
- 2 tablespoons poppy seeds
- 1 teaspoon organic baking powder
- 3 large organic eggs
- ¼ cup heavy cream
- ¼ cup salted butter, melted
- 3 tablespoons fresh lemon juice
- 1 teaspoon organic vanilla extract

- 20–25 drops liquid stevia
- 2 teaspoons fresh lemon zest, grated finely

DIRECTIONS

Preheat the oven to 350°F.

Line 12 cups of a muffin tin with paper liners.

Add flour, flax meal, poppy seeds, Erythritol, and baking powder in a mixing bowl and mix well.

In another mixing bowl, add eggs, heavy cream, and butter, and beat until well combined.

Add egg mixture into flour mixture and mix until well combined and smooth.

Add lemon juice, organic vanilla extract, and liquid stevia, and mix until well combined.

Gently, fold in lemon zest.

Place the mixture into prepared muffin cups evenly.

Bake for approximately 18–20 minutes or until a wooden skewer inserted in the center comes out clean.

Remove muffin tin from oven. Let it cool onto a wire rack.

Carefully invert the muffins onto a wire rack to cool completely before serving.

Nutrition: 255 Calories 23g Fat 5g Protein

CONCLUSION

Women looking for a quick and effective way to shed excess weight, get high blood sugar levels under control, reduce overall inflammation, and improve physical and mental energy will do their best by following a ketogenic diet plan. But there are special considerations women must take into account when they are beginning the keto diet.

A Ketogenic Diet is something that you should be starting with today for a better lifestyle if you are over 50. The ketogenic diet is more common in women than in men because of all the benefits it provides for dealing with the symptoms of menopause. Women who are experiencing menopause, or have already experienced it, have a clear idea of the troubles that come along with it. Menopause leads to fatigue, irritability and also increases weight. But the keto diet can help in controlling your body weight and also improve your physical well-being. Not sure from where or how to start with keto?

Being 50 years old or more is not bad. It is how we handle ourselves in this age that matters. Most of us would have just moved on and dealt with things as they would have arrived. That is no longer the case. It is quite literally survival of the fittest.

Do not try to work toward the lean body that many men sport. It is best for the overall function that women stay at twenty-two to twenty-six percent body fat. Our hormones will function best in this range, and we can't possibly work without our hormones. Like gymnasts and extreme athletes, very lean women will find their hormones no longer function or function at a less than optimal rate. And remember that the ideal weight may not be the right weight for you. Many women find that they perform their best when they are at their happy weight. If you find yourself fighting with yourself to lose the last few pounds you think you need to lose to have the perfect body, it may not be worth it. The struggle will affect your hormone function. Carefully observing the keto diet will allow your hormones to stabilize and regulate themselves back to their pre-obesity normal function.

As a woman, you know that sometimes your emotions get the better of you. It is true with your body, as you well know, and can be a major reason, women find it extremely difficult to lose weight the way they want to lose weight. We have been led to believe that not only can we do it all but that we must do it all. It gives many women extreme levels of pressure and can cause them to engage in emotional eating. Some women might have lowered self-worth feelings and may not feel they are entitled to the benefits of the keto diet, and turning to food relieves the feelings of inadequacy that we try to hide from the world.

The keto diet is naturally lower in calories if you follow the recommended levels of food intake. It is not necessary to try to restrict your intake of calories even further. All you need to do is only to eat until you are full and not one bite more. Besides losing weight, the keto diet aims to retrain your body on how to work properly. You will need to learn to trust your body and the signals it sends out to readjust to a proper way of eating.

Do not give up now as there will be quite a few days where you may think to yourself, "Why am I doing this?" and to answer that, focus on the goals you wish to achieve.

Whether you want to stay active, lose weight, look and feel better, or any of that, keto is your solution and a way of life that will ensure you get all you need.

CPSIA information can be obtained
at www.ICGtesting.com
Printed in the USA
LVHW011216190221
679460LV00003B/117

9 781914 257537